General Anatomy and Osteology of Head and Neck

General Anatomy and Osteology of Head & Neck

Mahdi Hasan
MBBS, M.S., (Honours)
Ph.D., D. Sc., FAMS
FNASC, FICS, FNA
Recipient of Dr. B.C. Roy National Award
Hony Professor, Dept of Anatomy
CSM Medical University, Erstwhile K.G. Medical College, Lucknow

Prashant Pratap
Saraswati Dental College, Lucknow

I.K. International Publishing House Pvt. Ltd.
NEW DELHI • BANGALORE

Published by
I.K. International Publishing House Pvt. Ltd.
S-25, Green Park Extension
Uphaar Cinema Market
New Delhi - 110 016 (India)
E-mail: ik_in@vsnl.net

ISBN 978-81-907770-5-6

Published by Krishan Makhijani for I.K. International Publishing House Pvt. Ltd., S-25, Green Park Extension, Uphaar Cinema Market, New Delhi - 110 016 and Printed by Rekha Printers Pvt. Ltd., Okhla Industrial Area, Phase II, New Delhi - 110 020.

Preface

This book covers essentials of gross anatomy of head and neck leaving out minutia but highlighting aspects of clinical application. It is different from the books, available on this subject in India on many accounts. First, it includes not only gross anatomy but also relevant details of osteology which is crucial for conceptualizing anatomical relations. Also it embodies essentials of histology with emphasis on identification of histology slides with the help of differential diagnosis tabulated for easy assimilation. Essentials of embryology required for the first professional BDS has also been highlighted. Need was felt for inclusion of all these as well as anthrometry required by the students of dentistry for orthodontia. Deficiencies in the aforementioned areas were felt by the Co-author (Prashant Pratap) as a first year student who discussed the problem with his teacher and mentor (Mahdi Hasan) and this book is the result of unique student-teacher collaboration. It took around five years to complete this project, during this period the Co-author passed all Professional examinations with flying colours. Inputs from his experience of later years in the areas of oral pathology, oral surgery, prosthodontia, periodontia and orthodontia have enriched this book.

We are highly thankful to Dr. A. Halim for his permission to use some figures from his BDS book, recently published by I.K. International Publishing House Pvt. Ltd.

It is our earnest hope that the unique manner in which this book has evolved with focus on clinical applications will find favours with students of dentistry of India and neighbouring countries.

Mahdi Hasan
Prashant Pratap

Contents

OSTEOLOGY

HISTOLOGY

1

Scalp

DEFINITION

Scalp comprises soft tissues covering the vault of the skull.

EXTENT

Generally hair bearing area on the top of the head. More precisely, from before backward: eyebrows to the superior nuchal line, side to side from one zygomatic arch to another, though the epicranial aponeurosis is adherent to the temporal lines on either side.

LAYERS

Surgical layer 1

S = skin, thick and rich in hair and sebaceous glands
C = Connective tissues, dense, interlacing criss-cross septa enclosing small spaces occupied by blood vessels and nerves
A = Aponeurosis - epicranial aponeurosis (of occipito frontalis muscle) also called galea (helmet) aponeurotica

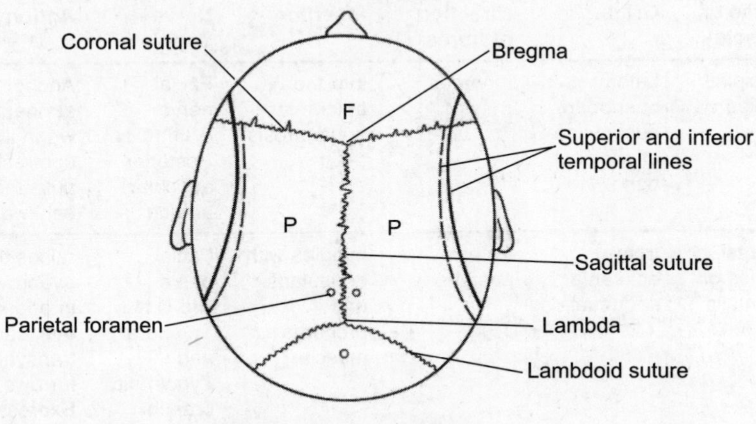

Fig. 1.1. Norma verticalis.

Surgical Layer 2

L = Loose areolar tissue layer, **danger layer**, wide and extensive, anteriorly runs to the eyelids deep to orbicularis oculi, posteriorly limited by the attachment of occipitalis to superior nuchal line.

Surgical Layer 3

P = Pericranium: periostium of cranial bones, dips at sutures, limited to the extent of the bone.

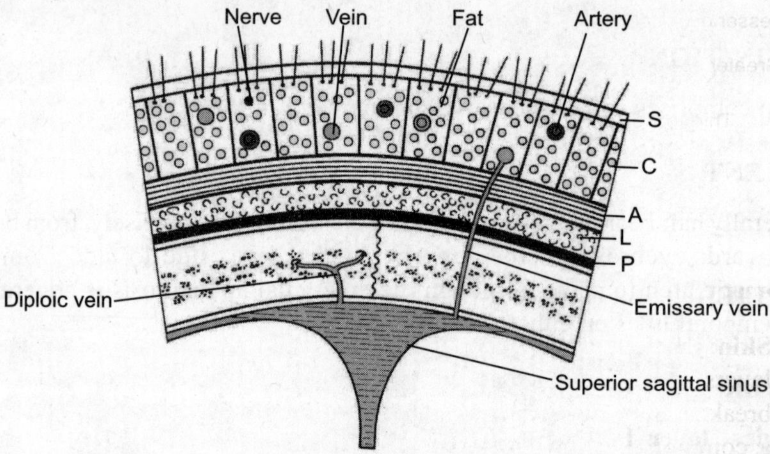

Fig. 1.2. Layers of scalp.

Muscles and aponeurosis—Occipito frontalis muscle, two occipital and two frontal bellies connected by the epicranial aponeurosis on the vertex (top of the skull)

Name of Muscle	Origin	Direction of fibres	Insertion	Nerve Supply	Action
Occipital bellies	Lateral ½ of superior nuchal line of occipital bone	forwards	into the epicranial aponeurosis	Facial nerve (VIIth C.N.) Posterior auricular branch	Anchors the aponeurosis, when it contracts it pulls the scalp backwards
Frontal bellies or Frontalis	from epicranial aponeurosis	Antero-posteriorly	mingles with orbicularis and procerus muscle	Facial nerve (VII C.N.) Temporal and Zygomatic branch	raises the eyebrows, helps in opening the eye, causes transverse furrows. Expression of surprise.

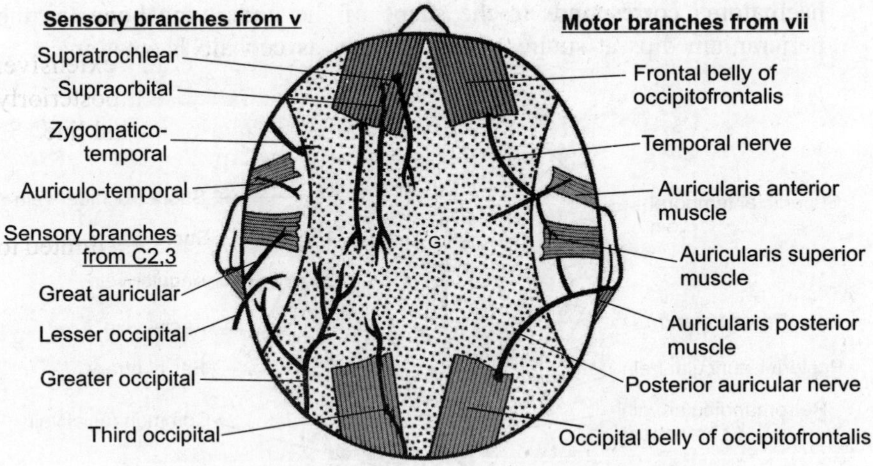

Fig. 1.3. Muscle and nerves of scalp.

APPLIED ANATOMY OF SCALP

1. **Skin:** Rich in hair, very strong. If caught in machinery, the first 3 layers of the scalp come out (avulsion of scalp) but the hair, do not break. Plenty of sebaceous glands are present in the scalp, hence it is a common site for development of sebaceous cysts.
2. **Dense Connective tissues:** Binds skin to the galea by criss-cross septa, containing blood vessels and nerves. Blunt injury causes localised accumulation of blood, (haematoma) which is very painful (due to rich nerve supply of scalp). If a cut or open wound occurs profuse bleeding occurs as the cut blood vessels are not able to retract (due to the adherence to the fibrous septa). Local pressure against the bone or a tourniquet (band) tied around the head (just above the level of the eyebrow is required to arrest the bleeding (as blood vessels to scalp come from periphery-centripetally).
3. If galea aponeurotica is cut in the coronal plane, the wound gapes (margins are pulled apart by the occipital and frontal bellies in the long axis of scalp.
4. Bleeding in loose areolar tissue layer causes a mobile haematoma (which can be pushed forward towards the eyes or backwards) extensive collection of blood occurs which gravitates to eyelids, leading to black eye after a few hours.
5. Bleeding deep to pericranium, commonly occurs in newborn babies after difficult childbirth (where a narrow pelvis compresses the large head of the baby during childbirth cephalo-pelvic disproportion). This

haematoma corresponds to the shape of the underlying bone (as the pericranium dips at sutures). it is known as cephalo haematoma.

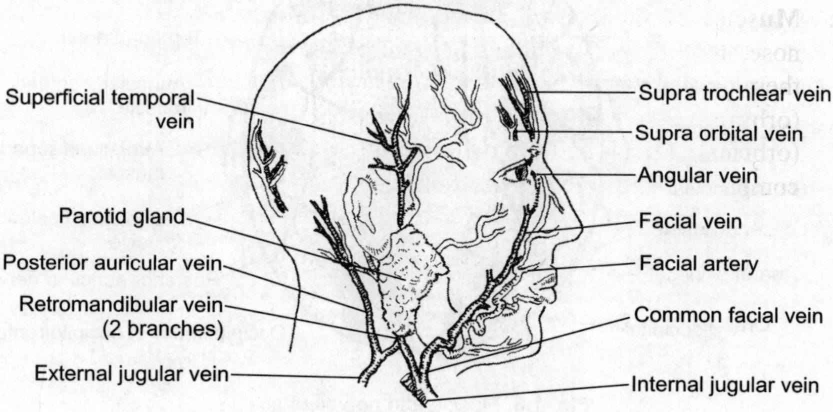

Fig. 1.4. Shows venous drainage of scalp and face.

FACE

Extent: Vertically from hairline to chin, horizontally from ear to ear. Thus forehead is common to both the face and scalp.

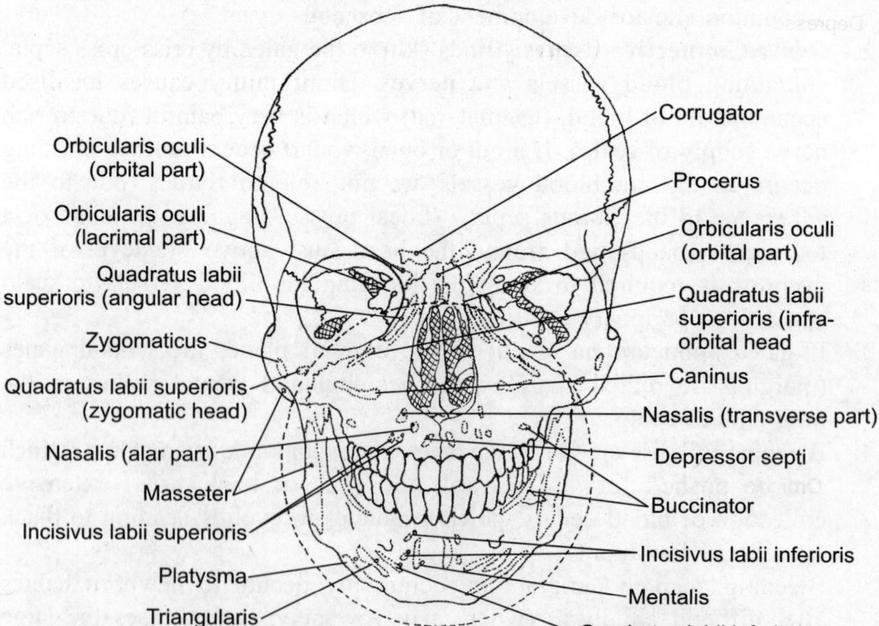

Fig. 1.5. Depicts sites of attachments of muscles of face.

1. **Skin:** Thin (thinnest skin of body is found in the eyelids) adherent to muscles (which insert into it and move the skin) (note: there is no deep fascia in the face.
2. **Muscles of face:** They are grouped around apertures of face (orbit, nose, mouth) and regulate or control the opening (either narrowing them—sphincter or enlarge the apertures—dilators). Muscle encircling (orbiting), the orbit and oral fissure are called orbicularis muscles (orbicularis oculi and orbicularis oris) around the nasal aperture are the compressor and dilator naris muscles.

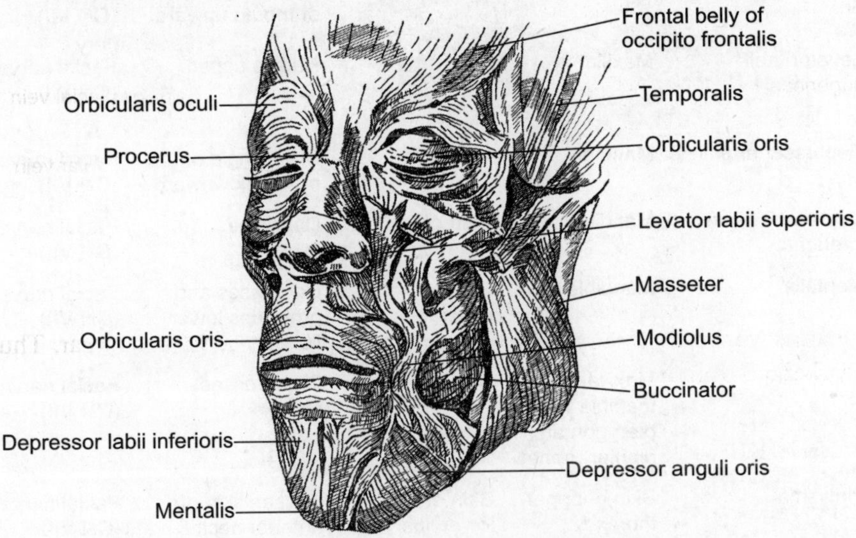

Fig. 1.6. Diagram showing muscles of face.

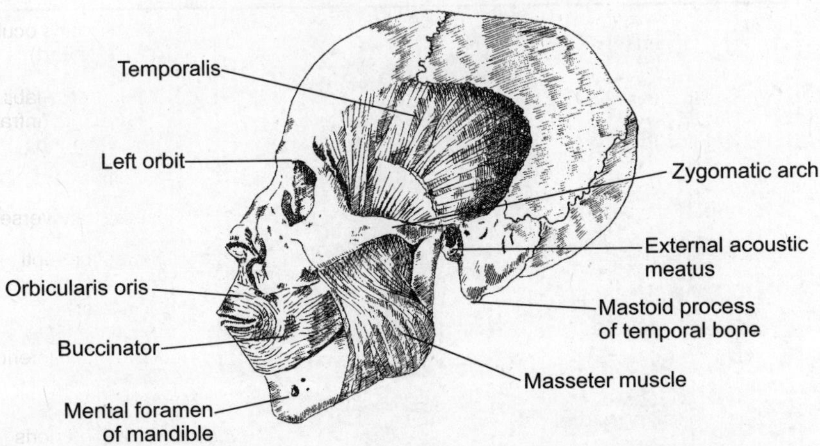

Fig. 1.7. Diagram showing the lateral side of the skull with its muscle attachments.

Table 1.1. Major Muscles of Facial Expression (arranged around orifices of face)

Orific	Origin	Insertion	Action	Innervation
Mouth (Oral Orifice)				
Orbicularis oris	Modiolus	Skin of lips	Close lips	Facial
Zygomaticus major	Zygomatic bone	Modiolus	Draws angle of mouth upwards	Facial nerve (CN VII)
Zygomaticus minor	Zygomatic bone	Skin of upper lip	Raises upper lip	Facial nerve (CN VII)
Levator anguli oris	Maxilla	Modiolus	Draw angle of mouth upward	Facial nerve (CN VII)
Levator labii superioris	Maxilla	Skin of upper lip	Raises upper lip	Facial nerve (CN VII)
Depressor anguli oris	Mandible	Modiolus	Draw angle of mouth downward	Facial nerve (CN VII)
Depressor labii inferioris	Mandible	Skin of lower lip	Depresses lower lip	Facial nerve (CN VII)
Mentalis	Mandible	Skin of lower lip	Depresses and protrudes lower lip	Facial nerve (CN VII)
Buccinator	Maxilla, manible and pterygoman dibular raphe	Skin of lips	Compresses cheeks	Facial nerve (CN VII)
Platysma	Skin of upper thorax & shoulder	Skin of lower lips & modiolus	Tenses skin of anterior neck & depresses lower lip & angle lip & angle of mouth	Facial nerve (CN VII)

2
Triangle of the Neck

TRIANGLES OF NECK

A single muscle mass in foetal life is longitudinally split into 2 muscles the (1) sternocleidomastoid anteriorly and the (2) trapezius posteriorly divides the quadrilateral area of the side of the neck into two triangles, an anterior and a posterior.

The boundaries of the anterior triangle are, in front, the median line of neck; above, the lower border of the body of the mandible, and an imaginary line drawn from the angle of the mandible to the sternocleidomastoid; behind, the anterior border of the sternocleidomastoid. The apex of the triangle is at the upper border of the sternum. The boundaries of the posterior triangle are,

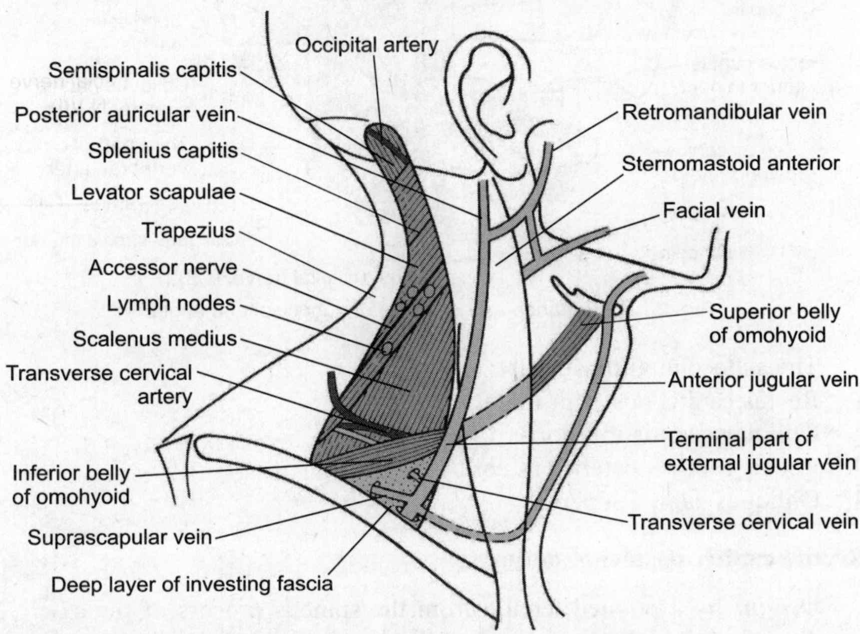

Fig. 2.1. Muscles in the floor of posterior triangle and contents—inferior belly of omohyoid and external jugular vein with tributaries.

in front, the posterior border of the sternocleidomastoid; below, the middle third of the clavicle; behind, the anterior margin of the trapezius. The apex corresponds with the meeting of the sternocleidomastoid and trapezius on the occipital bone. The anatomy of these triangles will be more fully described with that of the vessels of the neck.

Floor: is formed by

1. posterior atlanto-occipital membrane,
2. posterior arch of the atlas.
3. Vertebral artery and
4. First cervical nerve (or suboccipital nerve).

Nerve supply: The deep muscles of the back and the suboccipital muscles are supplied by the posterior primary divisions of the spinal nerves.

Contents

1. Third part of the vertebral artery.
2. Dorsal ramus of the nerve C1 (suboccipital nerve).
3. Suboccipital plexus of veins.

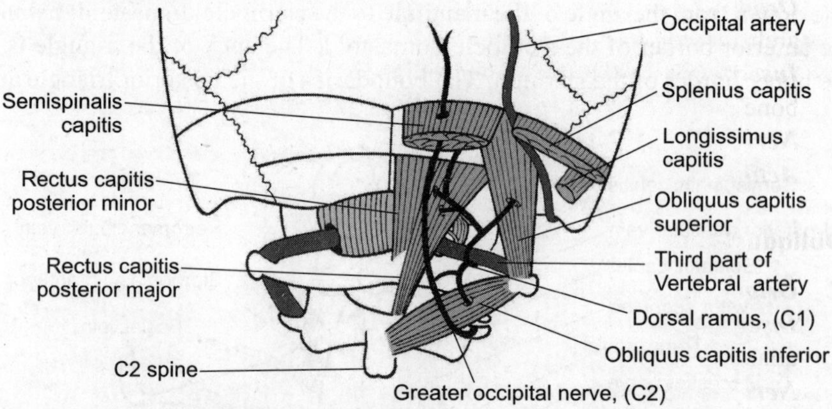

Fig. 2.2. Boundaries and contents of suboccipital triangle.

The suboccipital muscle are:

1. Rectus capitis posterior major,
2. Obliquus capitis inferior,
3. Rectus capitis posterior minor,
4. Obliquus capitis superior.

Rectus capitis posterior major

Origin: by a pointed tendon from the spinous process of the axis.
Insertion: into the lateral part of the inferior nuchal line of the occipital bone and the surface of the bone immediately below the line.

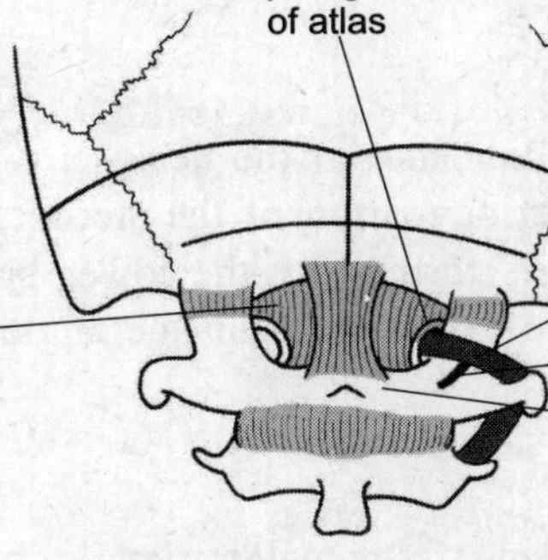

Fig. 2.3. Floor of suboccipital triangle.

Nerve supply: suboccipital nerve (C1)
Action: it rotates the skull along with the atlas, around the odontoid process, turning the face to the same side.

Rectus capitis posterior minor

Origin: by a narrow pointed tendon from the tubercle on the posterior arch of the atlas.
Insertion: into the medial part of the inferior nuchal line of the occipital bone and the surface between it and the foramen magnum.
Nerve supply: suboccipital nerve (C1)
Action: it extends the head

Obliquus capitis inferior: it is the larger of the two oblique muscles.

Origin: from the apex of the spinous process of the axis.
Insertion: into the lower and back part of the transverse process of the atlas.
Nerve supply: suboccipital nerve (C1)
Action: rotates the atlas, and with it the skull, around the odontoid process, turning the face to the same side.

Obliquus capitis superior

Origin: by tendinous fibers from the upper surface of the transverse process of the atlas, joining with the insertion of the preceding.
Insertion: into the occipital bone, between the superior and inferior nuchal lines, lateral to the semispinalis capitis.
Nerve supply: suboccipital nerve (C1)
Action: draws the head backward and to its own side.

ANTERIOR TRIANGLE

Boundaries

Anteriorly: by the median like of the neck
Posteriorly: by the anterior margin of the sternocleidomastoid;
Base: directed upward is formed by the lower border of the body of the mandible, and a line extending from the angle of the mandible to the mastoid process;
Apex: is below, at the sternum.

This space is subdivided into four smaller triangles by the digastric above, and the superior belly of the omohyoid below.

These smaller triangles are named the muscular, the carotid, the digastric, and the submental.

Subdivision of the anterior triangle of the neck are as follows:

1. Submandibular triangle
2. Carotid triangle
3. Muscular triangle
4. Submental triangle

1. MUSCULAR TRIANGLE

Boundaries

Anteriorly: by the median line of the neck from the hyoid bone to the sternum;
Posteriorly: by the anterior margin of the sternocleidomastoid;
Above: by the superior belly of the omohyoid.
Roof: skin, superficial fascia, platysma, and deep fascia, ramifying in which are some of the branches of the supraclavicular neves.
Floor: the sternohyoid and sternothyroid, which, together with the anterior margin of the sternocleidomastoid, conceal the lower part of the common carotid artery.

This vessel is enclosed within its sheath, together with the internal jugular vein and vagus nerve; the vein lies lateral to the artery on the right side of the neck, but overlaps it below on the left side; the nerve lies between the artery and vein, on a plane posterior to both. In front of the sheath are a few descending filaments from the ansa hypoglossi; behind the sheath are the inferior thyroid artery, the recurrent nerve, and the sympathetic truck; and on its medial side, the oesophagus, the trachea, the thyroid gland, and the lower part of the larynx. By cutting into the upper part of this space, and slightly displacing the sternocleidomastoid, the common carotid artery may be tied below the omohyoid.

2. CAROTID TRIANGLE

Boundaries

Posteriorly: by the sternocleidomastoid;
Inferiorly: by the superior belly of the omohyoid;
Superiorly: by the stylohyoid and the posterior belly of the digastric;
Roof: Skin, superficial fascia which contains platysma, and branches of the facial and cutaneous cervical nerves neck investing layer of the deep cervical fascia;
Floor: is formed by parts of the thyrohyoid, hyoglossus, and the middle and inferior constrictor of pharynx.

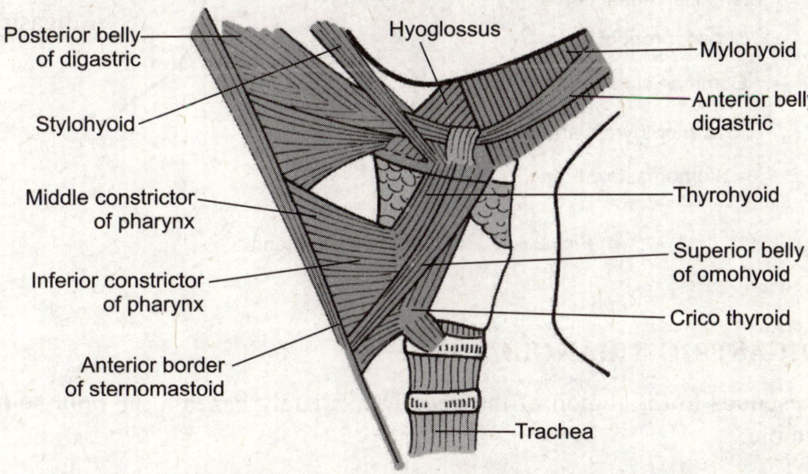

Fig. 2.4. Carotid triangle—boundaries and floor.

Contents: This space contains the upper part of the common carotid artery. Which bifurcates opposite the upper border of the thyroid cartilage into the external and internal carotid arteries. The following branches of the external carotid (1) the superior thyroid; (2) the lingual; (3) the facial; (4) the occipital, (5) ascending pharyngeal, are seen.

The nerves in this space are the following. The hypoglossal nerve crosses both the internal and external carotids above, curving around the origin of the occipital artery. With the sheath, between the artery and vein, and behind both, is the vagus neves; behind the sheath, the sympathetic truck. On the lateral side of the vessels, the accessory nerve runs for a short distance before it pierces the sternocleidomastoid; and on the medial side of the external carotid, just below the hyoid bone, may be seen the internal branch of the superior laryngal nerve; and, still more inferiorly, the external branch of the same nerve.

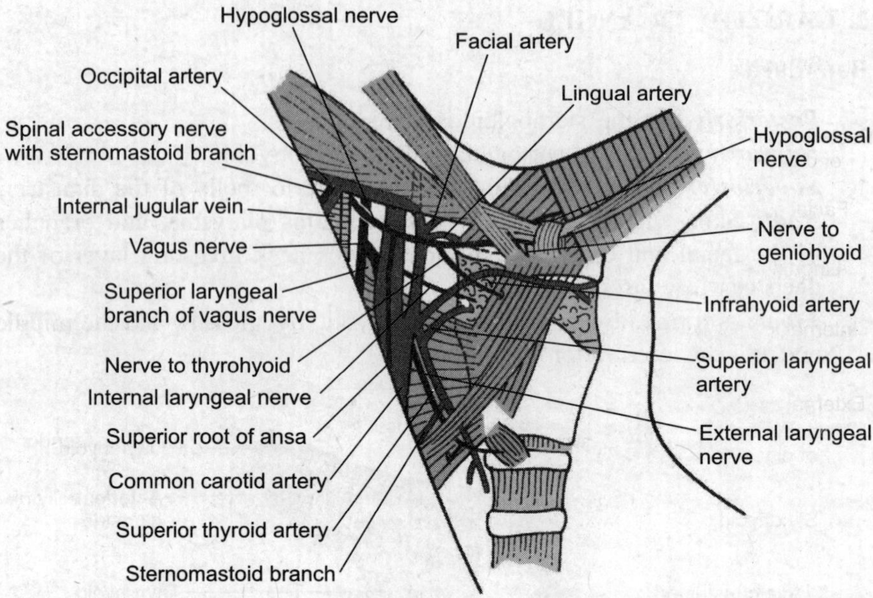

Fig. 2.5. Carotid triangle—contents.

3. DIGASTRIC TRIANGLE

Corresponds to the region of the neck immediately beneath the bofy of the mandible.

Boundaries

Above: the lower border of the body of the mandible, and a line drawn from its angle to the mastoid process;
Below: the posterior belly of the digastric and the stylohyoid;
Anteriorly: the anterior belly of the digastric.
Roof: by the skin, superficial fascia containing platysma, cervical branch of the facial nerve, the ascending branch of the transverse cutaneous nerve of the neck and deep fascia, and deep fascia which splits to enclose the submandibular gland.
Floor: is formed by the mylohyoid muscle anteriorly, hyoglossus posterioly, and superior and a small part of the middle constrictor of pharynx. It is divided into an anterior and a posterior part by the stylomandibular ligament. Anterior part contains the submandibular gland.

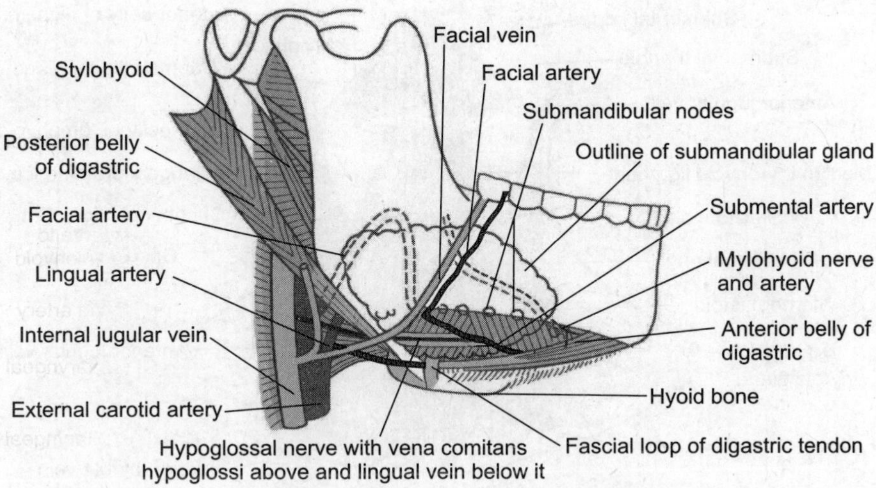

Fig. 2.6. Digastric triangle—contents.

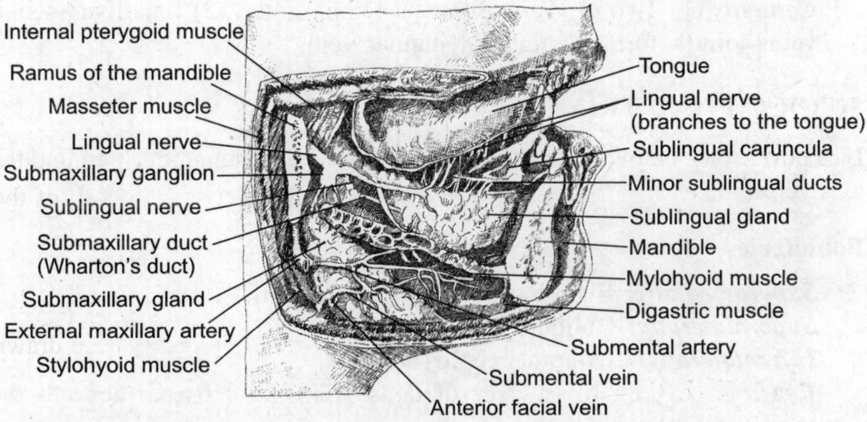

Fig. 2.7. Diagram showing the submandibular region.

4. SUBMENTAL TRIANGLE

Boundaries

Posteriorly: by the anterior belly of the digastric;
Anteriorly: by the median line of the neck between the mandible and the hyoid bone;
Below: the body of the hyoid bone;
Floor: is formed by the mylohyoid.

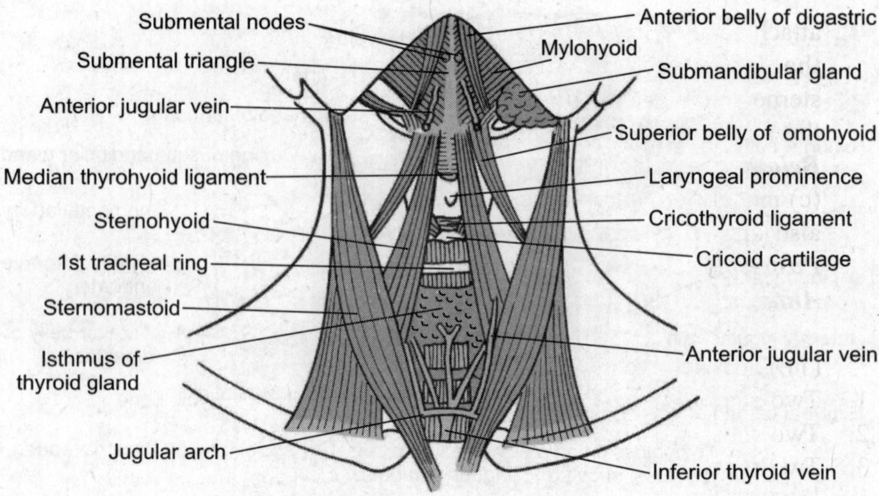

Fig. 2.8. Submental and muscular triangles and anterior median region of neck.

Contents (1) Two to four submental lymph nodes (2) Small submental veins join to form the anterior jugular vein.

SUBOCCIPITAL TRIANGLE

Lies posteriorly below the occipital bone, between its squamous part and the axis vertebra.

Boundaries

Superomedially: Rectus capitis posterior major;
Superolaterally: Obliquus capitis superior;
Inferolaterally: Obliquus capitis inferior.
Roof: is covered by a layer of dense fibro-fatty tissue, beneath the semispinalis capitis.

Fascia Colli (deep cervical fascia)

The fascia colli lies under cover of the platysma, and invests the neck like a muffler; it also forms sheaths for the carotid vessels.

Investing Layer

Attachments: Above to the (a) superior nuchal of the occipital bone, (b) mastoid process of the temporal bone, and (c) to the whole length of the inferior border of the body of the mandible. It splits to enclose the submandibular salivary gland and the deeper layer ascends up to attach to the mylohyoid line. (d) Opposite the angle of the mandible the fascia is very strong, and binds the anterior edge of the sternocleidomastoid firmly to that bone. (e) Between the mandible and the mastoid process it splits to enclose the parotid gland.

Below: It is attached to the (a) acromion process, (b) clavicle, and the (c) manubrium sterni. The fascia splits to enclose the suprasternal space also known as space of Burns; and the supraclavicular space.

Posteriorly: (a) Ligamentum nuchae (b) spine of 7th cervical vertebra.

Anteriorly: (a) symphysis menti (b) Hyoid bone .

(1) Thus the investing layer splits to enclose:

1. Two salivary gland (parotid + submandibular)
2. Two muscles (sternocleidomastoid + trapezius)
3. Two spaces (suprasternal + Supraclavicular)

(2) Carotid sheath encloses:

1. Common and internal carotid artery
2. Internal jugular vein
3. Vagus neve

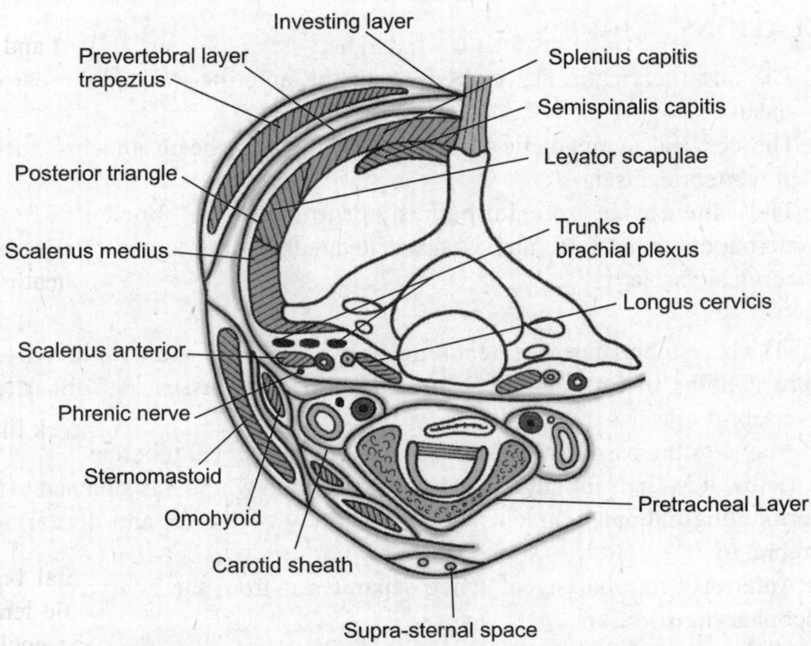

Fig. 2.9. Cervical fascia—transverse disposition of the three layers.

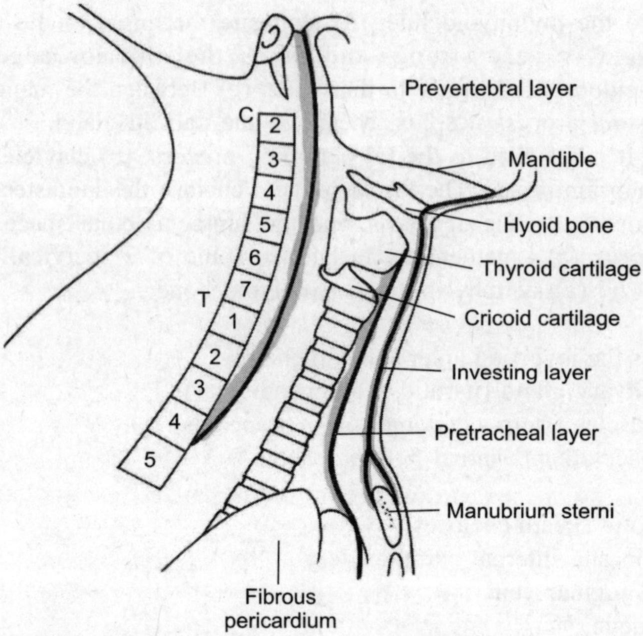

Fig. 2.10. Cervical fascia—vertical disposition of the three layers.

RELATIONS

1. The ansa cervicalis lies embedded in the anterior wall of the carotid sheath.
2. The cervical sympathetic chain lies behind the sheath attached to the prevertebral fascia.
3. The sheath is overlapped by the anterior border of the steronocleidomastoid, and is fused to all the three layers of the deep cervical fascia.

(3) Prevertebral fascia extends medialward behind the carotid vessels. where it helps in forming the carotid sheath, and passes in front of the prevertebral muscles.

Above to the base of the skull behind the pharyngeal tubercle.

Below it extends into the superior mediastinum where it is attached to the anterior longitudinal ligament and to the body of the 3rd and 4th cervical vertebra.

Anteriorly retroharyngeal space separates it from the pharynx and the buccopharyngeal fascia.

(4) Pretrachial fascia extends medially from investing layer in front of the carotid vessels, and assists in forming the carotid sheath. It continues

behind the depressor muscle of the hyoid bone, and, after enveloping the thyroid gland, prolonges in front of the trachea to meet the corresponding layer of the opposite side.

Above (a) oblique line of thyroid cartilage; and (b) cricoid cartilage (c) it is fixed to the hyoid bone.

Below the thyroid gland it encloses the inferior thyroid veins, passes behind the brachiocephalic vein, and finally behind with the arch of aorta. This layer is fused on either side with the prevertebral fascia, and with it completes the visceral compartment containing the larynx and trachea, the thyroid gland, and the pharynx and oesophagus.

Sternocleidomastoid (sternomastoid muscle) passes obliquely the side of the neck. It is thick and narrow at its central part, but broader and thinner at either end. It arises from the sternum and clavicle by two heads. The medial or sternal head is rounded and tendinous and arises from the upper part of the anterior surface of the mandubrium sterni, and is directed upward, lateralward, and backward. The lateral or clavicular head, composed of fleshy and of the medial third of the clavicle; it is directed almost vertically upward. The two heads are separated from one another at their origins by a triangular interval called sedilotts but gradually blend, below the middle of the neck, into a thick, rounded muscle which is inserted, by the strong tendon, into the lateral surface of the mastoid process, from its apex to its superior border, and by a thin aponeurosis into the lateral half of the superior nuchal line of the occipital bone.

French anatomists divide this muscle into four parts:

1. Sternomastoid
2. Sterno-occpitals
3. Cliedomastoid
4. Cliedo-occpitalis

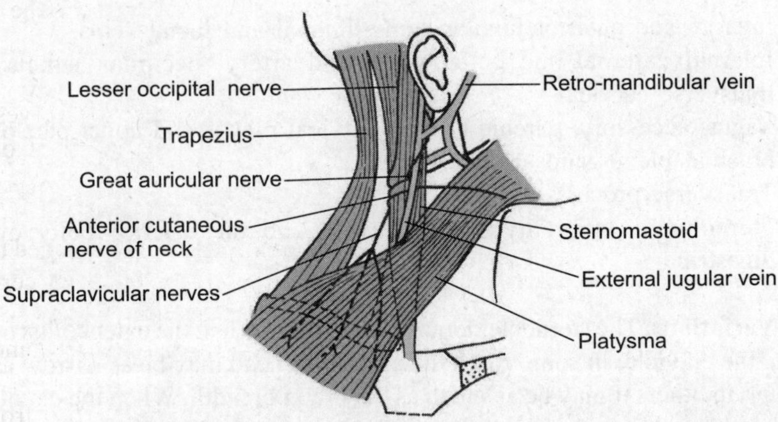

Fig. 2.11. Sternomastoid—superficial relations.

DIAGRAM

Nerve Supply

1. Spinal part of accessory nerve (purely motor) XI C.N.
2. C2 + C3 (mixed)

Actions

When only one sternocleidomastoid acts, it draws the head towards the shoulder of the same side. At the same time it rotates the heads so as to carry the face towards to opposite side. Acting together from their sternoclavicular attachments the muscles will flex the cervical part of the vertebral column, and extend the head on the neck as if looking over the shoulder of someone in a crowed. It the head is fixed, the two muscles assist in elevating the thorax in forced inspiration.

RELATIONS

Superficial

1. Skin.
2. Superficial fascia.
3. Playtysma.
4. External jugular vein and superficial cervical lymph nodes lying along the vein.
5. Transverse cutaneous nerve of neck.
6. Deep fascia.
7. Parotid gland overlaps the muscle.

Deep

1. Internal and anterior jugular veins, lingual and facial veins.
2. Internal external and common carotid artery; occipital, subclavian, transverse cervical.
3. Vagus, accessory, phrenic nerves; cervical plexus and upper part of the brachial plexus and ansa cervicalis.
4. Transverse process of atlas.
5. Sternohyoid, sternothyroid, omohyoid and the osterior belly of the digastric.

Variations. The sternocleidomastoid varies much in the extent of its origin from the clavicle; in some cases the clavicular head may be as narrow as the sternal; in others it may be as much as 7.5 cm in breadth. When the clavicular origin is broad, it is occasionally subdivided into several slios, separated by narrow intervals. More rarely, the adjoining margins of the sternocleidomastoid

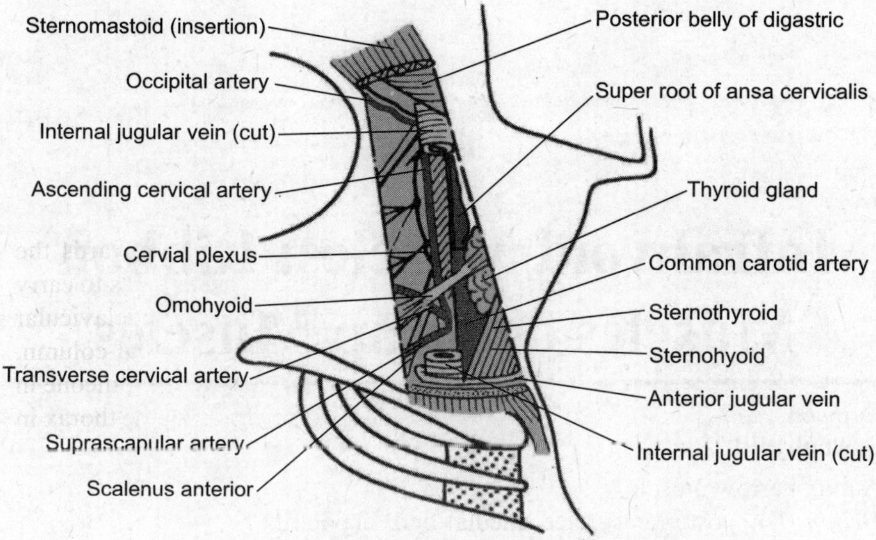

Fig. 2.12. Sternomastoid—deep relations.

and trapezius have been found in contact. The supraclavicular muscle arises from the manubrium behind the sternocleidomastoid and passes behind the sternocleidomastoid to the upper surface of the clavicle.

Table 2.1. Muscles of the Anterior Triangle.

Muscle	Origin	Insertion	Action	Innervation
Superficial musculature				
Sternocleidomastoid	Mastoid process of temporal bone	Sternum & clavical	Rotates head to opposite side & flexes neck	Spinal accessory n. (CN X)

3

Infrahyoid Muscles: Ribbon Muscles or Strap Muscles

Sternohyoid

A thin, narrow muscle

Origin: (i) posterior surface, medial end, clavicle,
(ii) posterior sternoclavicular ligament, and
(iii) upper and posterior part of the manubrium sterni

Direction of fibres: passing upwards and medially
Insertion: into the lower border, body of hyoid bone.
Nerve Supply: Ansa cervicalis (C1-2-3)

Sternothyroid

Sternothyroid is shorter, wider than sternohyoid beneath which it is situated.

Origin: Posterior surface of manubrium sterni, below sternohyoid, and the edge of the cartilage of first rib.
Direction of Fibres: upward and medialward.
Insertion: Oblique line on lamina of thyroid cartilage.
Nerve Supply: Ansa cervicalis (C1-2-3).
Action: Depresses larynx after elevation in swallowing and speech.

Thyrohyoid

Thyrohyoid small, quadrilateral muscle appearing like an upward continuation of sternothyroid.

Origin: oblique lien on lamina of thyroid cartilage,
Direction of Fibres: Upward and medial ward
Inserted: Lower border of greater cornu of hyoid
Nerve Supply: C1, through hypoglossal nerve
Action: Depresses hyoid. Also helps in elevating the larynx when hyoid is fixed by suprahyoid muscles.

Omohyoid

Omohyoid consists of 2 fleshy bellies united by a central tendon.

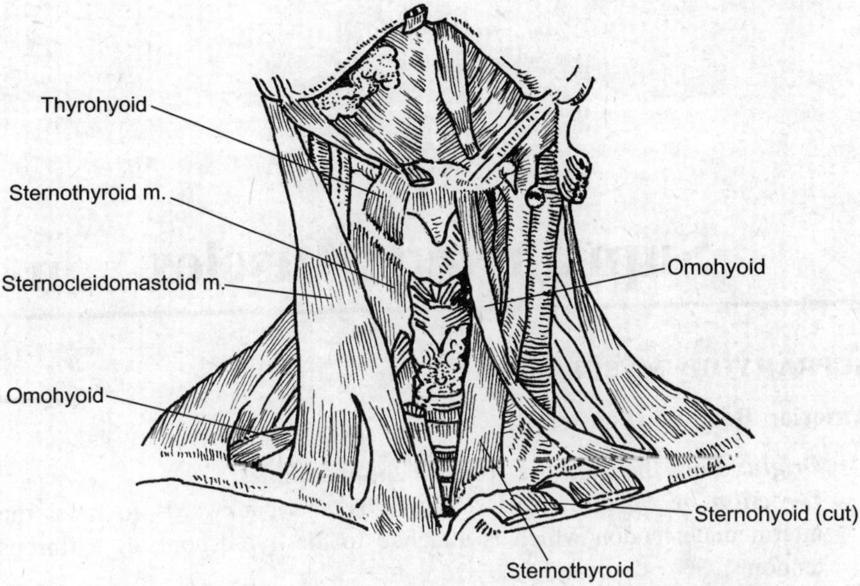

Fig. 3.1. Diagram showing sternocleidomastoid on right side and infrahyoid muscles on the left side.

Origin: from upper border of the scapula, and occasionally from superior transverse ligament which crosses the scapular notch.
Direction of Fibres: medially and upward
Insertion: Lower border of body of hyoid, lateral to sternohyoid
Nerve supply: Superior + Inferior roots of ansa cervicalis
Action: Depresses hyoid bone following its elevation during swallowing or speaking.

Table 3.1. Muscles of the Anterior Triangle

Muscle	Origin	Insertion	Action	Innervation
Infrahyoid musculature				
Geniohyoid	Anterior mandible	Hyoid bone	Protracts hyoid	Superior ramus of ansa cervical is (C1-C2)
Sternohyoid	Sternum	Hyoid bone	Lower hyoid	Superior ramus of ansa cervical is (C1-C2)
Thyrohyoid	Hyoid bone	Thyroid cartilage	Raises larynx	Superior ramus of ansa cervical is (C1-C2)
Sternothyroid	Sternum	Thyroid cartilage	Lower larynx	Superior ramus of ansa cervical is (C1-C2)
Omohyoid	Scapular notch	Hyoid bone	Lower hyoid	Superior ramus of ansa cervical is (C1-C2)

4

Suprahyoid Muscles

SUPRAHYOID MUSCLES

Anterior Belly of Digastric

Origin: from the digastric fossa of the mandible
Direction of fibre: it runs downwards and backwards to meet the intermediate tendon which is attached to the hyoid bone by a fibrous tendon.
Insertion: Into the intermediate tendon
Nerve Supply: Mylohyoid nerve branch of mandibular nerve
Action: It helps in depressing the mandible when the mouth is opened widely or against resistance; it also helps in elevating the hyoid bone, when mandible is fixed.

Posterior belly of Digastric

Origin: from the mastoid notch of the temporal bone
Direction of Fibre: It runs downwards and forwards to meet the intermediate tendon which is attached to the hyoid bone by a fibrous tendon
Insertion: Into the intermediate tendon
Nerve Supply: Facial nerve
Action: It helps in depressing the mandible when the mouth is opened widely or against resistance; it also helps in elevating the hyoid bone, when mandible is fixed (mouth is closed)

RELATIONS

Superficial

1. Mastoid process with the sternocleidomastoid muscle, the splenius and the longissimus capitis
2. The stylohyoid muscle
3. The parotid gland with the retromandibular vein

4. Submandibular salivary gland and lymph nodes
5. Angle of the mandible with the medial pterygoid

Deep

1. Transverse process of the atlas with the superior oblique and the rectus capitis lateralis
2. Internal and external carotid, lingual, facial and occipital arteries
3. Internal jugular vein
4. Vagus, accessory and hypoglossal nerve
5. Hypoglossal muscle

Borders

1. Upper border is related to the posterior auricular artery and the stylohyoid muscle
2. Lower border is related to the occipital artery

STYLOHYOID

Origin: arises from the posterior surface of the styloid process
Insertion: attached at the junction of the body and the greater cornu of the hyoid bone
Nerve Supply: Facial nerve
Action: it pulls the hyoid bone backwards and upwards and also helps in fixing the hyoid bone with the help of other muscle attached to the hyoid bone

MYLOHYOID

Origin: from the mylohyoid line on the inner surface of the mandible
Insertion: anterior and middle fibres are inserted into a median raphe which joins the right and left muscles; the posterior fibres are inserted into the body of the hyoid bone
Nerve supply: mylohyoid muscle
Action: it helps in elevating the floor of the mouth during the first stage of deglutition and also helps in the depression of the mandible and the elevation of the hyoid bone.

The 2 mylohyoid muscles emanate in midline and form oral diaphragm.

RELATIONS

Superficial platysma, anterior belly of digastric, submandibular salivary gland, mylohyoid nerve and vessels, submental branch of facial nerve, suprahyoid branch of lingual artery.

Deep hyoglossus, lingual nerve, submandibular ganglion, deep portion of submandibular gland and duct, hypoglossal nerve, communicating loop between lingual and hypoglossal nerve, vein accompanying hypoglossal nerve, geniohyoid muscle and the styloglossus muscle.

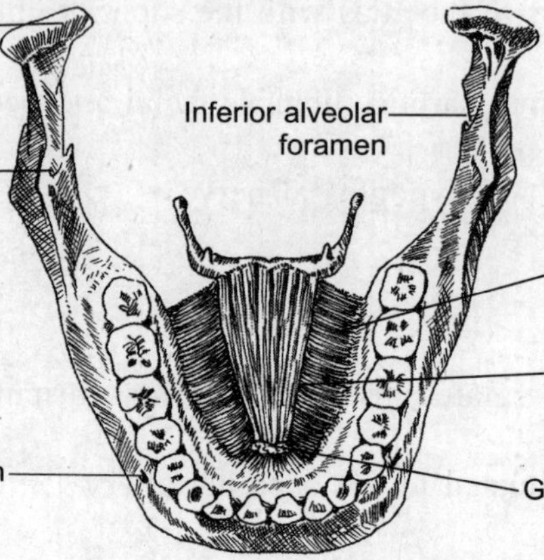

Fig. 4.1. Show superior surface of the two myclohyoid muscles forming oral diaphragm and 2 genioglosi in its oral surface.

GENIOHYOID

Origin: from the inferior genial tubercles (mental spine) of the mandible
Insertion: the fibres run backwards and downwards and are inserted into the anterior surface of the body of the hyoid bone
Nerve supply: the first cervical nerve—the fibres of the muscle pass through the hypoglossal nerve but it does not supply the muscle
Action: it helps in elevating the hyoid bone and also helps in depressing the mandible when the hyoid bone is fixed

Table 4.1. Muscles of the Anterior Triangle

Muscle	Origin	Insertion	Action	Innervation
Suprahyoid musculature				
Digastric:				
Posterior belly	Mastoid process of temporal bone	Anterior belly through hyoid throchlea	Elevates hyoid bone Facial n. (CN VII)	
Anterior belly	Posterior belly	Mandible		Mylohyoid branch of inferior alveolar n. (CN V3)
Mylohyoid	Body of mandible	Midline raphe	Elevates Floor of mouth & tounge	Mylohyoid branch of inferior alveolar n. (CN V3)
Styloyoid	Styloid process	Lesser horn of hyoid	Elevates & retracts hyoid	Facial n. (CN VII)

5
Muscles of the Eyeball

Four Recti Muscle (rectus = straight)

1. Superior rectus
2. Inferior rectus
3. Medial rectus
4. Lateral rectus

2 Oblique Muscle

1. Superior oblique
2. Inferior oblique

Nerve Supply of these muscles

Superior oblique muscle is supplied by the trochlear nerve (4th cranial nerve)
Lateral rectus muscle is supplied by the abducens nerve (6th cranial nerve)
All other muscles are supplied by the occulomotor nerve (3rd cranial nerve).

This can be remembered by the formula $SO_4 LR_6 AO_3$

SO_4- Superior oblique is supplied by the trochlear nerve which is the 4th cranial nerve

LR_6- Lateral rectus is supplied by the abducens nerve which is the 6th cranial nerve

AO_3- all other muscles (inferior oblique, superior rectus, inferior rectus, medial rectus) are supplied by the oculomotor nerve which is the 3rd cranial nerve.

Superior Oblique

Origin: from the body of the sphenoid, superomedial to the optic canal

Insertion into the sclera behind the equator of the eyeball, between the superior and the lateral rectus.

Inferior Oblique

Origin: from the orbital surface of the maxilla, lateral to the lacrimal groove. It is situated near the anterior margin of the orbit.

Insertion close to the superior oblique a little below and posterior to the later.

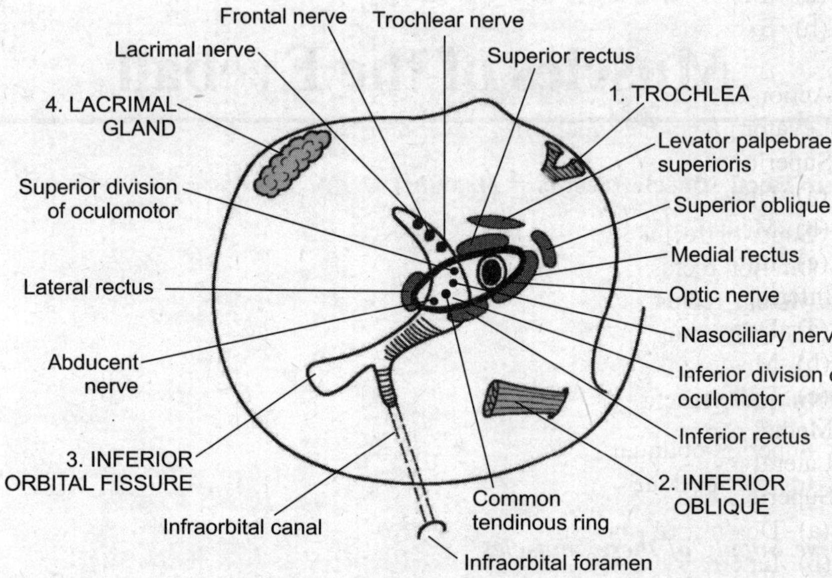

Fig. 5.1. Orbital muscles—origin; structures conducted through superior orbital fissure; one feature each at the four corners of orbit 1 to 4.

4 RECTI MUSCLE

Origin: from a common tendinous ring which is attached to the orbital surface of the apex of the orbit. It encloses the optic canal and the middle part of the superior orbital fissure.The lateral rectus has an additional small tendinous head which arises from the orbital surface of the greater wing of the sphenoid bone lateral to the tendinuous ring. ***Insertion:*** is into the sclera, a little posterior to the limbus. The average distances of the insertion from the cornea are:

Superior-7.7mm
Inferior- 6.5mm
Medial- 5.5mm
Lateral- 6.9mm

Action: The movement of the eyeball are as follows:

1. Around a transverse axis
   (a) Upward rotation or elevation (33 degrees)

(b) Downward rotation or depression (50 degrees)

2. Around a vertical axis
   (a) Medial rotation or adduction (50 degrees)
   (b) Lateral rotation or adduction (50 degrees)
3. Around an anteroposterior axis
   (a) Intortion
   (b) Extortion

Action of individual muscles:

1. Levator palpebrae superioris: elevation of upper eyelid
2. Superior rectus
   (a) Upward rotation
   (b) Medial rotation
   (c) Intortion
3. Inferior rectus
   (a) Downward rotation
   (b) Medial rotation
   (c) Extortion
4. Medial rectus: Medial rotation
5. Lateral rectus: Lateral rotation
6. Superior oblique
   (a) Downward rotation
   (b) Lateral rotation
   (c) Intortion
7. Inferior oblique
   (a) Upward rotation
   (b) Lateral rotation
   (c) Extortion

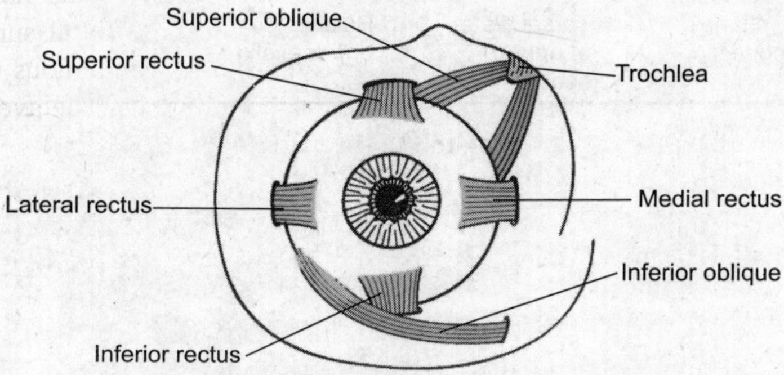

Fig. 5.2. Orbital muscles—insertion of recti.

Single pure movement of the eyeball:
Adduction: or movement towards the midline by the medial rectus, the superior and the inferior rectus
Abduction: or movement away from midline by the lateral rectus, by the superior and the inferior oblique.
Elevation: or upward movement by the superior rectus and the inferior oblique
Depression: or downward movement by the inferior rectus and the superior oblique
Extortion: by the inferior oblique and the inferior rectus
Intortion: by the superior oblique and the superior rectus

Table. Extraocular Muscles

Muscle	Origin	Insertion	Primary Action	Secondary Actions	Innervation
Superior rectus	Common tendinous ring for annulus tenderizes	Anterosuperior aspect	Elevation	Adduction & intortion	Oculomotor (CN III)
Inferior oblique	Maxilla	Posterolateral inferior quadrant	Elevation	Adduction & extortion	Oculomotor (CN III)
Inferior rectus	Common tendinous ring for annulus tenderizes	Anterosuperior aspect	Depression	Adduction & extortion	Oculomotor (CN III)
Superior oblique	Sphenoid bone	Posterolateral superior quadrant	Depression	Adduction & intortion	Trochlear (CN IV)
Medial rectus	Common tendinous ring for annulus tenderizes	Anteromedial aspect	Adduction		Oculomotor (CN III) Abducens (CN VI)
Lateral rectus	Common tendinous ring for annulus tenderizes	Anteromedial aspect	Adduction		Oculomotor (CN III)
Levator palpebrae superioris	Sphenoid bone	Tarsal plate of upper eyelid	Raises upper eyelid		

6

Temporomandibular Joint: Craniomandibular Joint

FEATURES TO BE NOTED

1. Bilateral joint (movement occurs simultaneously or concurrently in both right and left joint). No single joint can be moved alone. Both temporomandibular joints move as one unit.
2. Intra-articular disc—dense fibrous connective tissue (fibrocartilage).
3. It is a synovial type of joint.(Ginglymoarthrodial or hinge + plane type).

POINTS TO REMEMBER

1. Location – In front of tragus, below the zygomatic arch
2. Bones taking part – temporal bone articular eminence and mandible (condyloid process)
3. Articular surface – Articular eminence mandibular or glenoid fossa.
4. Type of joint – Synovial joint
5. Articular surface is covered by articular cartilage (fibrocartilage)
6. Disc or meniscus
7. Compartments of the joint
8. Fibrous capsule
9. Synovial membrane (lines the inner aspect of the capsule)
10. Ligaments – thickening of the capsule
11. Movements – Protraction, retraction, elevation, depression, side to side or chewing movement
12. Muscles taking part and their nerve supply
13. Nerve supply of joint
14. Arterial supply, venous drainage, lymphatic drainage
15. Applied importance or clinical anatomy.

INTRA-ARTICULAR DISC (OR MENISCUS)

Dense fibrous tissue which has elastic tissue posteriorly.It is thicker posteriorly, has upper and lower laminae. Sometimes there is a perforated central area

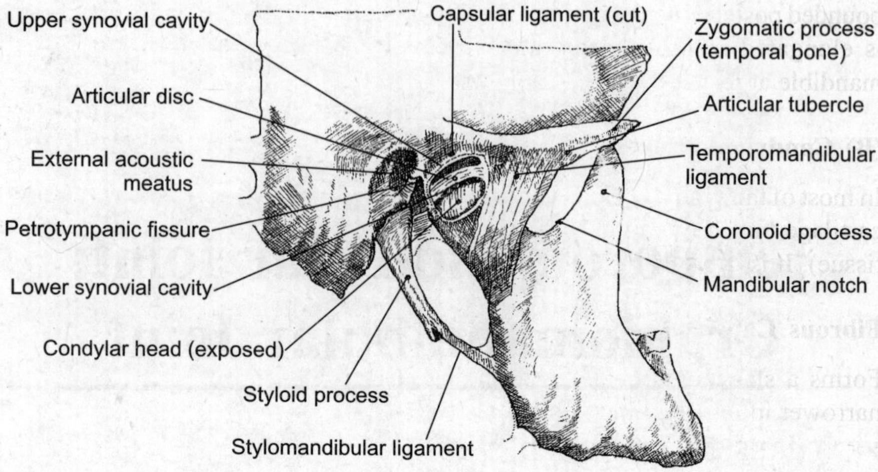

Fig. 6.1. Diagram showing the TMJ region.

which is very thin (about 1mm in thickness) anteriorly the disc is 2 mm in thickness and it is thickest posteriorly (about 3mm)

Superiorly: Concavo-convex
Inferiorly: Incongruent

Joint surface fitting together – congruent
Joint surface not fitting together – incongruent

Temporomandibular joint as such incongruent, but it is made congruent by the disc

FUNCTIONS OF THE DISC

1. To make the incongruent articular surfaces congruent, thus strengthening the joint.
2. To serve as a shock absorber or washer.
3. To facilitate proper spreading of synovial fluid and providing friction free movement.

ARTICULAR SURFACE

(A) Articular eminence, glenoid fossa (at rest)

Convexo-concave from before backwards and concave downwards. Articular eminence, which is a horizontal bar of bone or tubercle of the root of the zygoma, articular, is the main component during movement (glenoid fossa, bounded posteriorly by posterior glenoid tubercle and squamotympanic fissure is elongated mediolaterally and is occupied by the condyloid process of mandible at rest.

(B) Condyloid Process

In most of the synovial joints the articular surface is covered by hyaline (glassy) cartilage but in this joint there is an exception (it is made of dense fibrous tissue). It is fibro-cartilagenous, only a few cartilage cells can be seen.

Fibrous Capsule

Forms a sleeve and encloses the joint surface. Its is wider superiorly and narrower inferiorly, like a funnel.

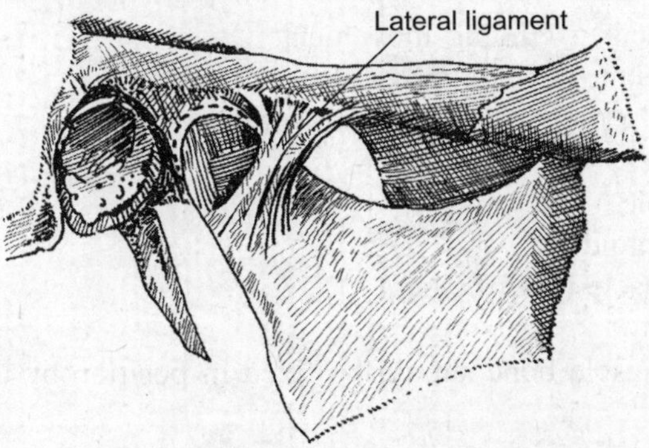

Fig. 6.2. Showing lateral aspect of temporomandibular joint.

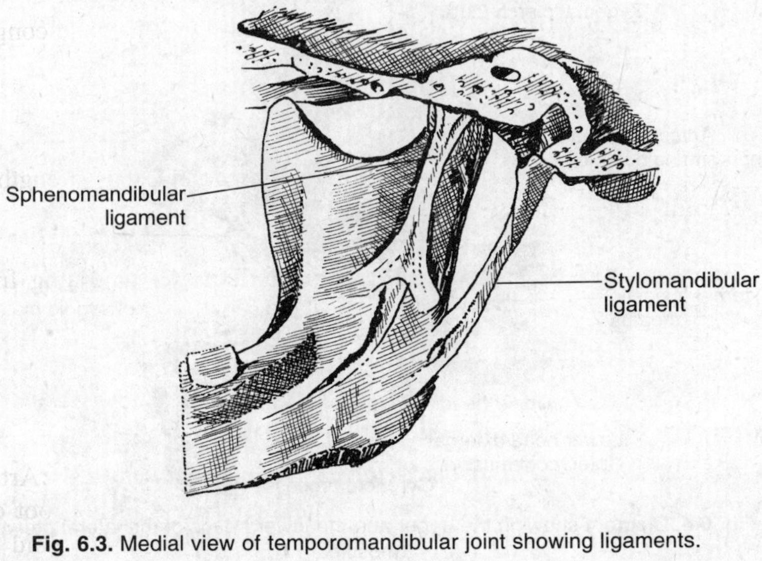

Fig. 6.3. Medial view of temporomandibular joint showing ligaments.

Synovial Membrane

It covers the inner aspect of the capsule and peripheral part of the disc but does not cover the articular cartilage covered areas.

Movement and Muscles

1. Opening of the mouth or depression of the mandible
2. Closing the mouth or elevation of the mandible.
3. Protraction (or protrusion) of mandible.
4. Retraction (or retrusion) of mandible.
5. Side to side, or chewing movement (2-3 mm space between the anterior teeth in resting position), maximum width when opened is about 3 finger bredth or 1.5 inches (4 cm).

Upper compartment = Gliding movement
Lower compartment = Hinge movement or rotation
Opening of the mouth (Complex movement)

Muscle couple
1. Lateral pterygoid
2. Digastric muscle (both bellies)

The hyoid muscle bone should be fixed in position by the infra-hyoid muscles namely:
1. Sternohyoid

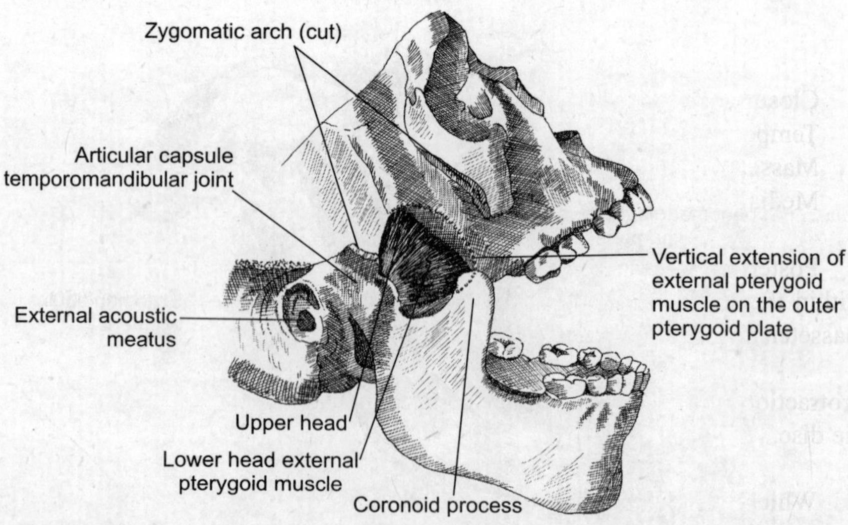

Fig. 6.4. Diagram showing the upper and the lower heads of the lateral pterygoid muscle.

2. Sternothyroid – Thyrohyoid
3. Omohyoid

Thereafter, the digastric muscle contracts and depresses the chin and pulls it downwards and backwards, causing opening of the mouth.

Lateral pterygoid muscle protracts the mandible and pulls the disc and the neck of the mandible forwards (due to the gliding movement in the upper compartment).

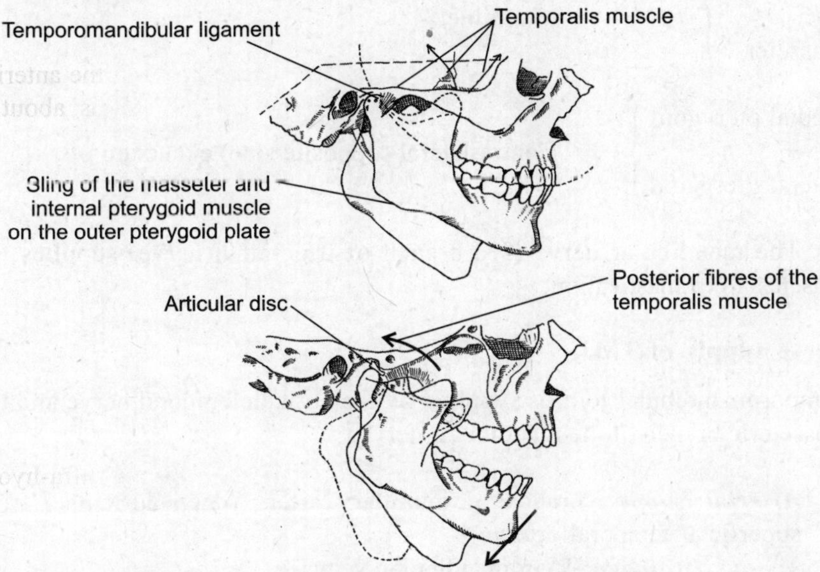

Fig. 6.5. Diagram showing movement of the mandible.

Closure of mouth or elevation of mandible by :

1. Temporalis
2. Masseter
3. Medial pterygoid

Posterior fibres of the temporalis first retracts the protracted mandible within the mandibular fossa, the anterior and middle fibres of temporalis, masseter, and medial pterygoid then elevate the mandible (or close the mouth).

Protraction of mandible in upper compartment between temporal bone and the disc.

Which muscles protract the mandible?

1. Lateral pterygoid.
2. Superficial fibres of masseter + medial pterygoid helps.

Retraction of mandible

Retraction of mandible in the upper compartment is done by posterior fibres of temporalis.

Side to side or chewing movement in both compartments (both lateral and medial pterygoid muscles of both sides acting alternately).

Temporalis + Masseter	Ipsi-lateral (same side) Mandible
Medial pterygoid + Lateral Pterygoid	Contra-lateral (opposite side) excursion of

The mandibular nerve (3rd branch of trigeminal nerve) supplies the muscles all of mastication.

Nerve supply of TMJ

Temporomandibular joint is supplied by the auriculotemporal nerve and the masseteric branch of the mandibular nerve.

Arterial Supply: branch of maxillary artery (deep auricular) from superficial temporal artery.
Venous Drainage: Retromandibular vein.
Lymphatic Drainage: Parotid lymph node.

RELATIONS

1. Laterally – skin, superficial fascia, deep fascia
2. Posteriorly – overlapped by the parotid gland and crossed by superficial temporal vessels and behind them the auriculotemporal nerve
3. Medially – anriculo temporal n., spine of sphenoid and chorda
4. Superiorly – middle cranial fossa and menings tympani n.
6. Anteriorly – lateral pterygoid muscle and masseteric nerve.

APPLIED ANATOMY

1. Clicking or popping sounds of the joint is caused because of the disorder of the disc (the disc lags behind and does not follow the condyloid process). A dental surgeon can listen to this sound by placing a stethoscope in front of the tragus and below the zygomatic arch.

2. Dislocation:
   (a) ***Anterior Dislocation:*** In a normal joint, while opening the mouth, the condyloid process is located below the articular eminence. In case of anterior dislocation, the head comes to lie in the inferior temporal fossa (the bone can be relocated by placing the thumb on the third molar and applying pressure downwards and then elevating the chin).
   (b) ***Posterior Dislocation:*** Posterior tympanic plate fractures can cause the condyloid process to lie in the external acoustic meatus, hence hindering the hearing capacity of the individual.
   (c) ***Central Dislocation:*** Of the mandibular fossa into the middle cranial fossa due to a jab in boxing or an accident. The condyloid process may rest in the middle cranial fossa (because the bone separating the middle cranial fossa and the condyloid process is very thin) the joint can be relocated by surgery.
   (d) ***Medial Dislocation:*** Fracture of the spine of sphenoid bone can cause hindrance in the nerve supply of the salivary glands by the auriculotemporal and chorda tympani nerve resulting in a marked reduction in the secretion of saliva causing dryness of the mouth.
3. The neck of the mandible is the weakest part and is the most common site of fracture.

Medial to the spine of sphenoid lies the chorda tympani nerve which supplies the following two salivary glands and carries taste from anterior 2/3rd of the tongue.

1. Submandibular gland
2. Sublingual gland

Lateral to the spine of sphenoid lies the auriculotemporal nerve which supplies the parotid gland.

Fracture of the spine of sphenoid in case of medial dislocation of TMJ causes damage to both chorda tympani and auriculotemporal nerves. Hence causing no secretion from all the major salivary glands resulting into dryness of the mouth.

Temporomandibular joint is a synovial, compound ginglymo arthrodial type of joint

Ginglymo – Hinge
Arthrodial – Plane
Gliding type – Upper compartment
Hinge type – Lower compartment

Infantile angle of mandible is about 170 degree and coronoid process is higher than condyloid process. Temporomandibular joint lies at the level of occlusal surface of teeth.

7
Muscles of Mastication

POINTS TO REMEMBER

1. Location
2. Shape
3. Parts
4. Development
5. Origin
6. Direction of fibres
7. Insertion
8. Arterial supply
9. Nerve supply
10. Venous drainage
11. Lymphatic drainage
12. Action
13. Relation
14. Type of movement
15. Applied anatomy

TEMPORALIS

Location: It is located on the lateral side of the skull.
Shape: fan-shaped muscle
Parts: It has 3 parts: anterior, middle and posterior
Origin: From the temporal fossa and the temporal fascia

Temporal fossa comprises:

1. Greater wing of sphenoid bone
2. Inferior half of parietal bone
3. Squamous part of temporal bone
4. Temporal surface of frontal bone

Insertion: into the coronoid process of mandible (apex, posterior border upto the depth of the mandibular notch Anterior border upto the retromolar fossa and the medial surface upto the temporal crest)

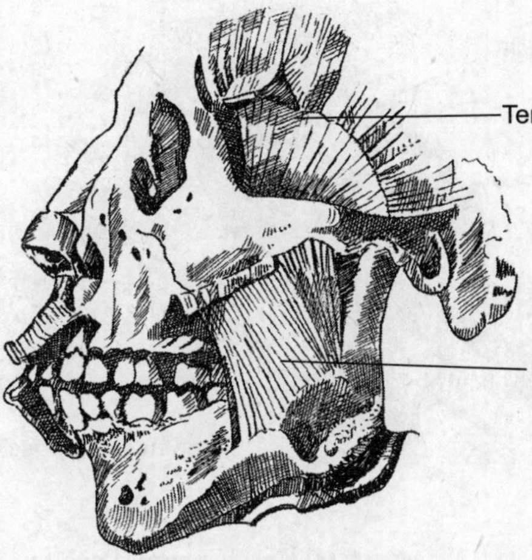

Fig. 7.1. Showing temporalis and masseter.

RELATIONS

Superficial: (a) Temporal fascia (b) Temporal branch of facial nerve (c) Epicranial aponeurosis (d) Auriculotemporal nerve (e) Auricular anterior and superior muscles (f) Superficial fascia of skin (g) Skin.

Deep: (a) Deep temporal nerves and vessels (b) Temporal fossa comprising 4 bones (Pterion).

Anterior: (a) Zygomatic bone (b) Zygomatico temporal nerve.

Actions: (a) Anterior and middle fibres elevate with masseter, medial pterygoid (b) Posterior fibres retract the protracted mandible.

Nerve Supply: It is supplied by the deep temporal branches of anterior division of mandibular nerve.

Arterial supply: Deep temporal branches of the maxillary artery.

Venous Drainage: Maxillary vein and retromandibular vein.

Lymphatic Drainage: Parotid lymph nodes and upper deep cervical lymph nodes.

Applied Anatomy: The tonus of the temporalis is responsible for the position of the mandible at rest when the intercuspid distance between the upper and lower incisor is 1-3 mm. It is an anti-gravity muscle. Hence, after death the gravity pulls the mandible downwards and the mouth remains open.

Development: 1st brachial arch mesoderm.

MASSETER

Location: Posterior part of face, in front of the ear (auricle) covered by the parotid gland and lies below by the zygomatic arch.

Shape: Quadrilateral

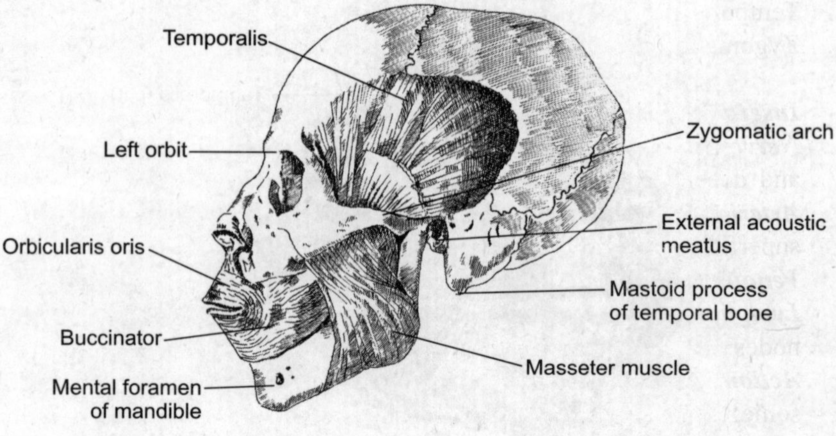

Fig. 7.2. Lateral view of skull showing masseter, temporalis and buccinator muscles.

Parts: Superficial, Middle and Deep

Origin: Anterior most fibres arise from zygomatic process of the maxilla and lower border of zygomatic arch

Middle fibres arise from the lower border of the middle 2/3rd of zygomatic arch.

Deep fibres arise from the medial surface of the middle 2/3rd of the zygomatic arch.

Zygomatic arch is made up of :

1. Zygomatic process of maxilla
2. Lower border of zygomatic bone

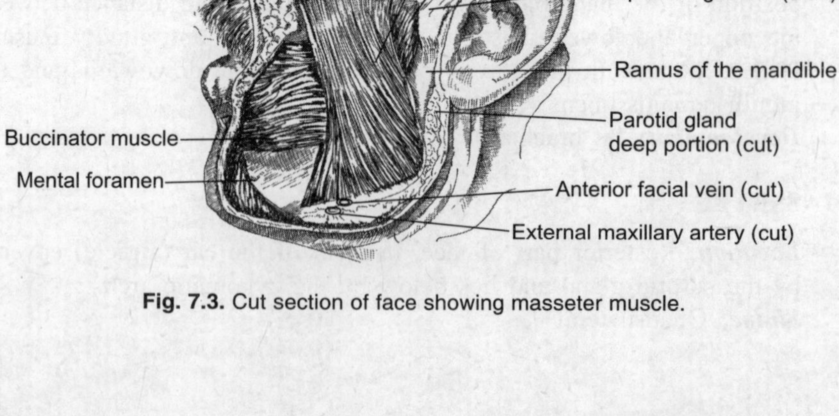

Fig. 7.3. Cut section of face showing masseter muscle.

3. Temporal process of zygomatic bone
4. Zygomatic process of temporal bone

Insertion: Ramus of mandible upto the level of the 2nd molar tooth
Nerve Supply: Masseteric nerve supplies it, and divides it into middle and deeper fibres
Arterial Supply: Masseteric artery (branch of maxillary artery), divides superficial from middle fibres of masseter
Venous Drainage: Maxillary vein and retromandibular vein,
Lymphatic Drainage: Parotid lymph nodes, upper deep cervical lymph nodes.
Action: Anterior fibres help in protraction with lateral pterygoid and to some extent, medial pterygoid. They are antagonist to posterior fibres of temporalis.The muscle as a whole elevates the mandible (closes the mouth) acting together with temporalis and medial pterygoid.

RELATIONS

Superficial: (a) Skin (b) superficial fascia (c) platysma (d) risorius (e) deep fascia, called parotidio masseteric fascia.
Anteroinferior: angle is crossed by facial vein and artery
Anterior: Buccal pad of fat and branches of facial nerve and parotid duct crosses.
Deep: (a) Ramus of mandible (b) temporalis muscle attached to coronoid process (c) buccinator muscle lies deep to it.

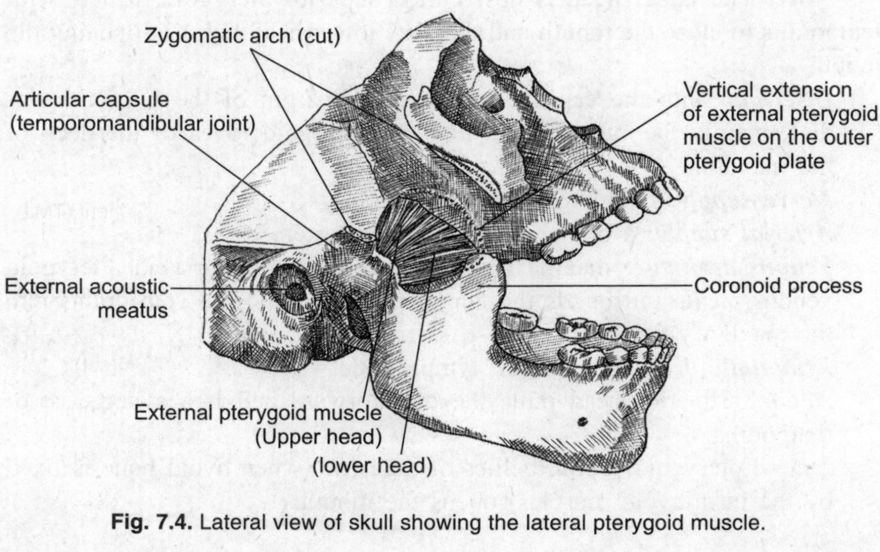

Fig. 7.4. Lateral view of skull showing the lateral pterygoid muscle.

APPLIED ANATOMY

1. It is responsible for pressing the teeth together,(or clenching the teeth) it is active when one is under stress, tension, or pain.
2. The muscle becomes very large hypertrophy in people who grind their teeth in sleep (Bruxism). A plastic guard is put on the teeth to protect them from wear and tear, and preventing erosion of the enamel.

   Electromyography: has shown that the upper fibres are active during closure of mouth. Hence it is also called superior pterygoid.

   Spasm: Can cause anterior dislocation of the mandible, which may be due to the epileptic fits or electroconvasive shock, given to a psychiatric patients.

LATERAL PTERYGOID

Location: The infra-temporal fossa. The infra-temporal crest separates the infra-temporal fossa from the temporal fossa.

Origin: (1) The upper head of lateral pterygoid arises from infra-temporal surface of the greater wing of sphenoid below the infra-temporal crest. (2) The lower head arises from the lateral surface of lateral pterygoid plate.

Fibres: The upper fibres are directed downwards and backwards in a transverse plane.

Lower fibres are elongated vertically near the lower triangular apex in the infra-temporal fossa.

Note: The upper head is now called superior pterygoid, it acts with temporalis to close the mouth and only the lower head helps in opening the mouth.

Insertion: into the capsule and anterior margin of the intra-articular disc, mainly the upper head, and the pterygoid fovea of the neck of the mandible.

Nerve supply: mandibular nerve.

Arterial supply: a branch from maxillary artery.

Venous drainage: maxillary vein and retromandibular vein. Pterygoid venous plexus surrounds the lateral pterygoid and the vein drains into the maxillary vein.

Lymphatic drainage: Parotid lymph node.

Action: Superior head pulls the disc forward and is a synergesist of temporalis.

Lateral pterygoid + both bellies of digastric (when hyoid bone is fixed by the infra-hyoid muscles) opens the mouth.

Lower head pulls the neck forward and helps in opening the mouth, but both the heads cause protraction of the mandible.

RELATIONS

Deep: (a) mandibular nerve exits through foramen ovale (b) accessory meningeal artery (c) middle meningeal artery (d) otic ganglion (e) tensor palati.

Superficial: (a) temporalis (b) zygomatic arch (c) coronoid process of mandible (d) partly masseter (d) deep fascia (e) superficial fascia (f) skin.

APPLIED ANATOMY

The lateral pterygoid muscle is surrounded by a plexus of vein called pterygoid plexus, which communicates with the facial vein through the deep facial vein and the cavernous sinus by emissary veins passing through foramen ovale.

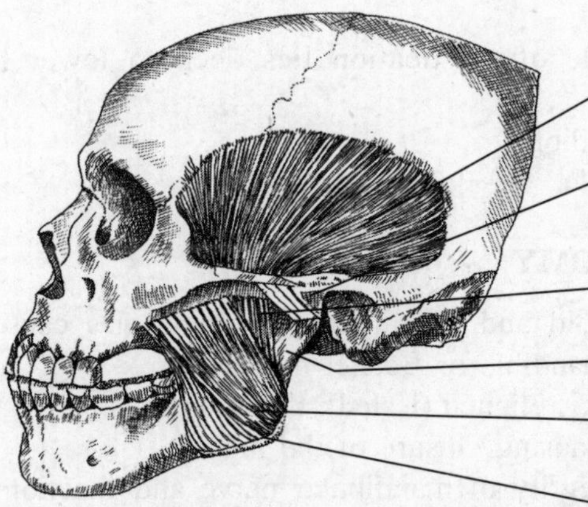

Fig. 7.5. Lateral view of skull showing temporalis and masseter muscles.

MEDIAL PTERYGOID

Location: Infratemporal fossa

Shape: Quadrilateral

Origin: (1) Deep fibres arise (mainly from sphenoid bone) from the medial surface of the lateral pterygoid plate and from pterygoid fossa.

2. Superficial head from :
   (a) Tuberosity of maxilla
   (b) Pyramidal process of palatine bone

Direction of fibres: downwards, backwards, and laterally.
Insertion: medial surface of the ramus of the mandible below the mandibular foramen. Anterior extent upto mylohyoid groove, inferior-going to lower border around the angle.
Nerve supply: From the trunk of mandibular nerve
Arterial supply: branches from maxillary artery
Venous drainage: Maxillary vein and retromandibular vein
Lymphatic drainage: Parotid lymph nodes

The nerve to medial pterygoid trunk of mandibular nerve passes through the otic ganglion but it does not relay there.

Actions: Elevation of mandible, along with masseter and temporalis, anterior fibres help in protraction.

Bennet movement (lateral) with lateral pterygoid.

Lateral and medial pterygoid are important for chewing or mastication.

RELATIONS

1. Deepest muscle of mastication lies deep to lower head of lateral pterygoid
2. Ramus of mandible
3. Masseter muscle.

APPLIED ANATOMY

1. Medial pterygoid and lateral pterygoid muscles cause contra-lateral excursion of mandible or Bennet movement.
2. When jaw jerk is elicited (tested), this muscle is active with temporalis and masseter causing closure of the mouth.
3. It tests the integrity of mandibular nerve and function of medial and lateral pterygoid.

In case of an injury to mandibular nerve, the chin is directed to the same side by the opposite pterygoid muscles when the mouth is opened. The chin deviates to the side of injury by the normal pterygoid muscles.

8

Paranasal Air Sinuses

NAMES

1. Maxillary
2. Frontal
3. Ethmoidal
4. Sphenoidal

MAIN FUNCTIONS

1. Air-conditioning – It warms the inspired air in winter and cools the inspired air in summer to equalise the temperature to around the normal body temperature and also controls the humidity. It does not allow the temperature of inspired air to be very high or very low.
2. Resonation of voice – It causes change in voice.

Classification

- **Anterior group**
  1. Maxillary
  2. Frontal
  3. Anterior ethmoidal
- **Posterior group**
  1. Posterior ethmoidal
  2. Sphenoidal

Openings of Paranasal Air Sinuses

- **Anterior group**
  - All open in the middle meatus of nose
- **Posterior group**
  - Posterior ethmoidal – Sphenoethmoidal recess
  - Sphenoid sinus – Superior meatus

Three shelf-like projections in lateral wall, called conchae or turbinates. Meatus is the part that lies between or below the concha.

Sphenoethmoidal Recess – above the superior concha (between sphenoid and ethmoid bone)

Development of all paranasal air sinuses from diverticular evagination from lateral wall of nose and they arise during fetal life except frontal and sphenoidal which arises after birth. The frontal air sinus arises in the 2nd year (frontal bone). Sphenoidal air sinus appears soon after 2nd year.

They have spurts of growth at the time of eruption of

1st molar		6-8 years.
2nd molar	post puberty	12-14 years

and thus they increase the height of the face from birth to puberty.

Maxillary Sinus (Antrum of Highmore)

It resembles a 4-sided pyramid with the apex directed laterally towards the zygomatic bone, base towards the lateral wall of nose medially, roof and superior wall into the floor of orbit and orbital plate of maxilla. The floor or inferior wall on the alveolar process of maxilla.

Alveolar process of maxilla (The roots of 2nd premolar and 1st molar projects into it, in case of a small sinus).

1st molar, 2nd molar, 1st premolar, 2nd premolar are located in the floor, (it can be confirmed with an x-ray).

Anterior surface – Facial surface

Posterior surface – related to pterygopalatime fossa.

Lateral wall of nose inferior concha, inferior meatus and high up in the middle meatus (below middle concha) is the normal ostium (opening of antrum)

Inferior concha – Separates cartilagenous bone

Superior and middle concha – are process of ethmoidal bone (not separate bone).

PROCESS

Zygomatic – lateral
Frontal – superamedial
Palatine – medial
Alveolar – inferior

Inferior Concha: A separate bone articulates with the base of maxilla. Below this concha lies inferior meatus.

Frontal Process: — Anterior-nose
— Posterior lacrimal
— Superior frontal

Alveolar process: Bears teeth of upper jaw

Palatine process: Anterior 3-4th of palatine process, horizontal plate of palatine bone (L-shape).

Nerve supply:

1. Anterior superior alveolar nerve
2. Inferior orbital nerve

Anterolaterally between the mucous membrane and the bone

Epithelium + connective tissue + mucous secreting glands

Facial artery, deep facial vein, runs below and other superficial muscle of face.

Posterior wall:

Pterygopalatine fossa – maxillary nerve and 3rd part of maxillary artery and vein.

Maxillary sinusitis – causes pain in 5th and 6th teeth in small sinuses and 4th to 7th teeth in case of large sinuses.

Infection of tooth – Abscess of tooth may cause pain in the maxillary sinus, because they are supplied by the same nerves and vessels.

Cancer – may extend to the floor of orbit and may cause increased pressure on the eyeballs resulting in the protrusion of the eyeball. The whole affected maxilla may have to be removed by an orofacial surgeon assisted by a plastic surgeon. This procedure is called maxillectomy.

Aeronautic Dentistry – A person who has got the first or second molar extracted should not fly immediately thereafter because perforation of sinus can occur due to the pressure changes at high altitude (because the molars are related to the maxillary sinus).

NERVES AND VESSELS

1. Anterior superior alveolar nerve and vessels
2. Middle superior alveolar nerve and vessels
3. Posterior superior alveolar nerve and vessels
4. Infra-orbital nerve and vessels

Lymphatic drainage by submandibular lymph nodes

The last air inhaled goes into the maxillary sinus and the 1st air exhaled is from this sinus because of its location.

FRONTAL SINUSES

Lies deep to the middle of the superciliary arch in the frontal bone. Sometimes it may extent into the orbital plate of frontal bone. (X-ray can be done to confirm this.)

Septum – The midline is usually deviated, its opening lies in the middle meatus through the frononasure tongue.

Nerve supply – Ophthalmic nerve (branch of trigaeminal nerve). Its frontal and supraorbital branches.

Arterial supply – Supra-orbital artery (branch of internal carotid artery).

Venous Drainage – Unites with the supratrochlear to form angular vein (at the medial angle of eye) continues as the facial vein.

Lymphatic Drainage – Submandibular lymph node.

Anterior Ethmoidal

Anterior part of labyrinth of ethmoid deep to media wall of orbit. The anterior ethmoidal opens in the anterior part of hiatus semilunaris of middle meatus below opening of frontal sinus.

Nerve Supply: Anterior ethmoidal nerve (nasociliary branch of ophthalmic nerve).

Arterial Supply: Anterior ethmoidal artery (branch of ophthalmic artery)

Venous Drainage: Anterior ethmoidal vein drains into ophthalmic vein.

Posterior Ethmodial

lies in the posterior part of labyrinth of ethmoid in medial wall of orbit (posterior part) and opens in superior meatus.

Nerve supply: Posterior ethmoidal nerve branch of nasociliary nerve, branch of ophthalmic nerve.

Arterial supply: Posterior ethmoidal artery branch of ophthalmic artery.

Venous Drainage: Posterior ethmoidal vein opens into inferior ophthalmic vein.

Lymphatic Drainage: Retropharyngeal lymph nodes.

Sphenoidal Sinus

Body of sphenoidal below the hypophyseal fossa between the two cavernous sinuses. It opens into the sphenoethmoidal recess.

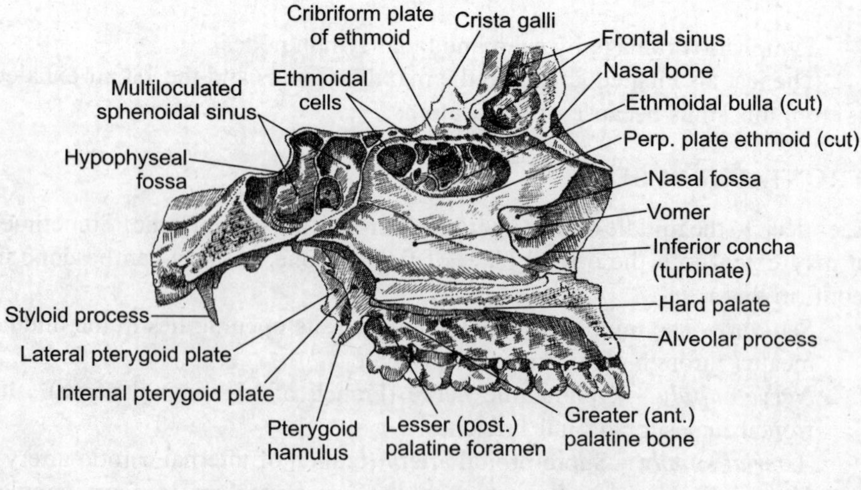

Fig. 8.1. Cross-section showing frontal sinus.

Nerve Supply: Posterior ethmoidal nerve, nasociliary branch of ophthalmic nerve.

Arterial Supply: Posterior ehtmoidal artery branch of ophthalmic artery, branch of internal carotid artery.

Venous Drainage: Posterior ethmoidal vein branch of inferior ophthalmic vein.

Lymphatic Drainage: Retropharyngeal lymph nodes.

Sinusitis: Inflammation of sinus causing pain in the region of the sinus

Frontal, maxillary, anterior ethmodial, anterior nasal drains mainly occur into the anterior nasal aperture.

Posterior nasal sinus – Nasal drip occurs and trickles down the throat and causes coughing.

9

Tongue

PAPILLAE OF TONGUE

1. **Vallate papillae**—also called circumvallate papillae. It is the largest of the papillae, lie just anterior to the foramen caecum and the sulcus terminalis.They are circular in outline and are surrounded by a trench or moat.They vary in number, averaging from around 8 to 12.
2. **Fungiform papillae**—they are more numerous in number and smaller in size and are found at the sides and the apex of the tongue. They can be recognized by their red colour and broader, rounded upper surface.They are non-keratinized.
3. **Filiform papillae**—thin hair like (keratinized) papillae which covers the anterior two third of the tongue they are more prominent in children and less in adults and are whitish in colour.
4. **Folliate papilla**—it is found mainly in rabbits, on the side of tongue, just anterior to sulcus terminalis.

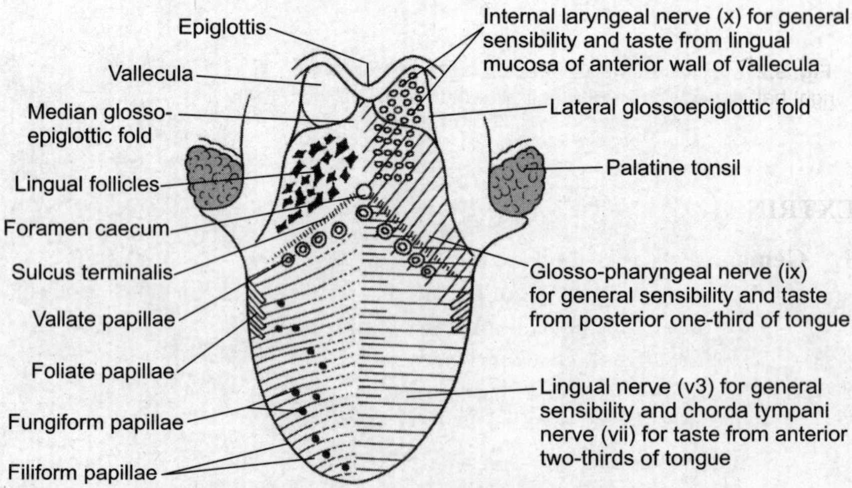

Fig. 9.1. Dorsum of the tongue showing papillae on right half and sensory nerve supply on left half.

MUSCLES OF TONGUE

Intrinsic Muscles

1. **Superior longitudinal** lies beneath the mucous membrane and shortens the tongue and makes its dorsum concave.
2. **Inferior longitudinal** lies close to the inferior surface of the tongue and shortens the tongue and makes its dorsum convex.
3. **Transverse** extends from the median septum to the margins and makes the tongue narrow and elongated.
4. **Verticalis** found at the borders of the anterior part of the tongue and makes the tongue broad and flattened.

Nerve supply—all intrinsic muscle are supplied by the hypoglossal nerve

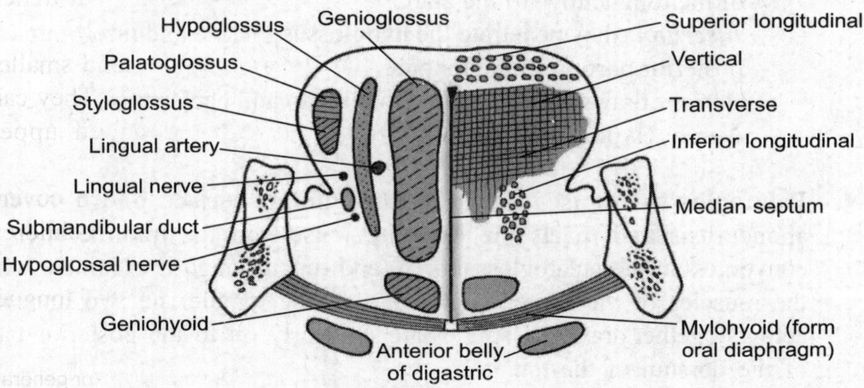

Fig. 9.2. Muscles of the tongue in a coronal section showing extrinsic muscles in the right half and intrinsic muscles in the left half. Note the mylohyoid muscle forming the floor of the mouth.

EXTRINSIC MUSCLES

1. **Genioglossus** is a thick paired muscle.
   - *Origin:* it arises from the mental spine (superior genial tubercles) of the mandible.The muscle extends backward and upward
   - *Insertion:* the lower fibres inserting into the hyoid bone and epiglottis.The bulk of the muscle spreads out through the body of the tongue toward the dorsum, intermingling with intrinsic muscle fibres.
   - *Action:* its action results into the drawing forward and downward of the tongue.
   - *Nerve:* Hypoglossal nerve.

2. **Hyoglossus** is flat and triangular. It lies medial to and above the submandibular gland and the mylohyoid muscle. Its fibres intermingle with the styloglossus muscle fibres.
   - ***Origin:*** is from the upper margin and the greater cornua of the hyoid bone.
   - ***Insertion:*** into the body of the tongue towards the apex.
   - ***Action:*** contraction of this muscle draws the tongue downward and backward.
   - ***Nerve:*** Hypoglossal nerve.

3. **Styloglossus** is long and narrow
   - ***Origin:*** on the styloid process and the stylohyoid ligament. It extends downward forward and medially to the outer surface of the hyoglossus muscle.Some of its fibres pass under the lateral margin of the tongue toward the apex.
   - ***Insertion:*** they penetrate the hyoglossus muscle and insert into the posterior portion of the tongue.
   - ***Action:*** draws the root of the tongue up and backwards.
   - ***Nerve:*** Hypoglossal nerve.

4. **Palatoglossus**—It is attached to the inferior surface of the palatal aponeurosis and meets the opposite muscle in the midline.Then it converges on the palatoglossal arch, and runs through it to mingle with the muscles of the posterolateral part of the tongue.The two muscles acting together,draw the soft palate inferiorly on to the posterior part of the dorsum of the tongue.

ARTERIAL SUPPLY

Lingual artery branch of external carotid artery.The root of the tongue is also supplied by the tonsillar branch of the ascending pharyngeal arteries.

VENOUS DRAINAGE

Two venae comitantes run with the lingual artery and are joined by the dorsal lingual vein. One vena comitans runs with the hypoglossal nerve.

LYMPHATIC DRAINAGE

Jugulomohyoid lymph node is called the main lymph node of the tongue. From the posterior part of the tongue it goes to the upper deep cervical lymph node. The tip of the tongue drains into the submental lymph node.

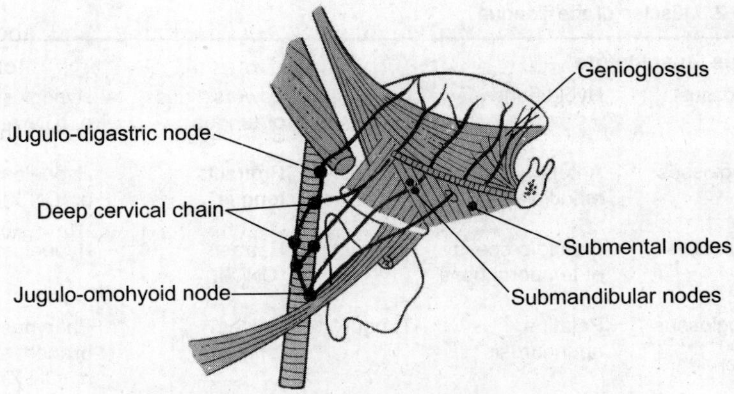

Fig. 9.3. The lymph drainage of the tongue.

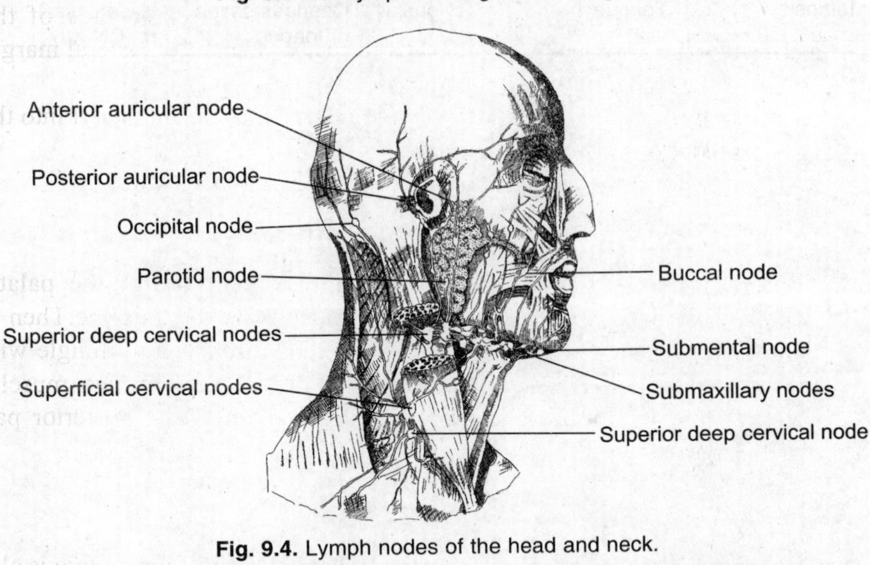

Fig. 9.4. Lymph nodes of the head and neck.

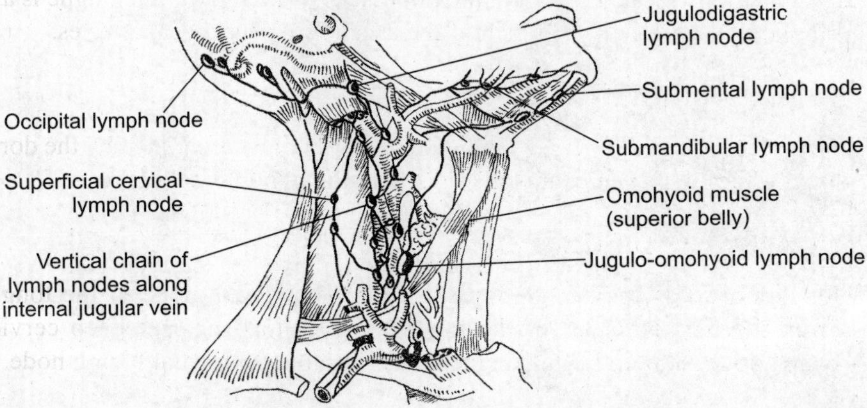

Fig. 9.5. Lymphatic drainage of neck.

Table 2. Muscles of the Tongue

Tongue Musculature				
Hyoglossus	Hyoid bone	Lateral tongue	Lowers sides of tongue	Hypoglossal n. (CN XII)
Genioglossus	Anterior mandible	Tongue	Protracts tongue	Hypoglossal n. (CN XII)
Styloglossus	Styloid process of temporal bone	Tongue	Retracts (CN XII)	Hypoglossal
Palatoglossus	Palatine aponeurosis	Tongue	Raises tongue	Pharyngeal branch, of vagus n. (CN X)
Intrinsics	Tongue	Tongue	Changes shape of tongue	Hypoglossal n. (CN XII)

10

Pharynx

Pharynx is that part of the digestive tube which is placed behind the nasal cavities, mouth, and larynx. It is a musculomembranous tube, and is conical in form, with the base upward, and the apex downward, extending from the under surface of the skull to the level of the cricoid cartilage in front, and that of the sixth cervical vertebra behind. The cavity of the pharynx is about 12.5 cm long, and broader transversely than antero-posteriorly in diameter. Its broadest part lies immediately below the base of the skull, where it projects on either side, behind the pharyngeal ostium of the auditory tube, as the pharyngeal recess; its narrowest point is at its termination in the oesophagus.

RELATION

Superiorly: By the body of the sphenoid bone and basilar part of the occipital bone.

Inferiorly: it is continuous with the oesophagus at the level of the 6th cervical vertebra.

Posteriorly: it is connected by loose areolar tissue with the cervical portion of the vertebral column, and the prevertebral fascia covering the longus colli and longus capitis muscles.

Anteriorly: it is incomplete, and is attached to the medial pterygoid plate, pterygomandibular raphe, mandible, tongue, hyoid bone, and thyroid and cricoid cartilages.

Laterally: it is connected to the styloid processes and their muscles, and is in contact with the common and internal carotid arteries, the internal jugular veins, the glossophayngeal, vagus, and hypoglossal nerves, and the sympathetic truncks. Seven cavities communicate with it e.g., the two nasal cavities, the two tympanic cavities, the mouth, the larynx, and the oesophagus.

The cavity of the pharynx may be subdivided from above downward into three parts: nasal, oral, and laryngeal.

Nasopharynx or the nasal part of pharynx lies behind the nose and above the level of the soft palate: it differs from the oral and laryngeal parts of the pharynx in that its cavity always remains patent. In front, it communicates through the conchae with the nasal cavities. On its lateral wall is the pharyngeal ostium of the auditory tube, somewhere triangular in shape, and bounded behind by a firm prominence, the torus or cushion, caused by the medial end of the cartilage of the tube which elevates the mucous membrane. A vertical fold of mucous membrane, the salpingopharyngeal fold, stretches from the lower part of the torus; it contains the salpingopharyngeus muscle. A second and smaller fold, the salpingopalatine fold, stretches from the upper part of the torus to the palate. Behind the ostium of the auditory tube is a deep recess, the pharyngeal recess. On the posterior wall is a prominence, best marked in childhood., produced by a mass of lymphoid tissue, which is known as the pharyngeal tonsil. Above the pharyngeal tonsil, in the middle line, an irregular flask-shaped depression of the mucous membrane sometimes extends up as far as the basilar process of the occipital bone; it is known as the pharyngeal bursa.

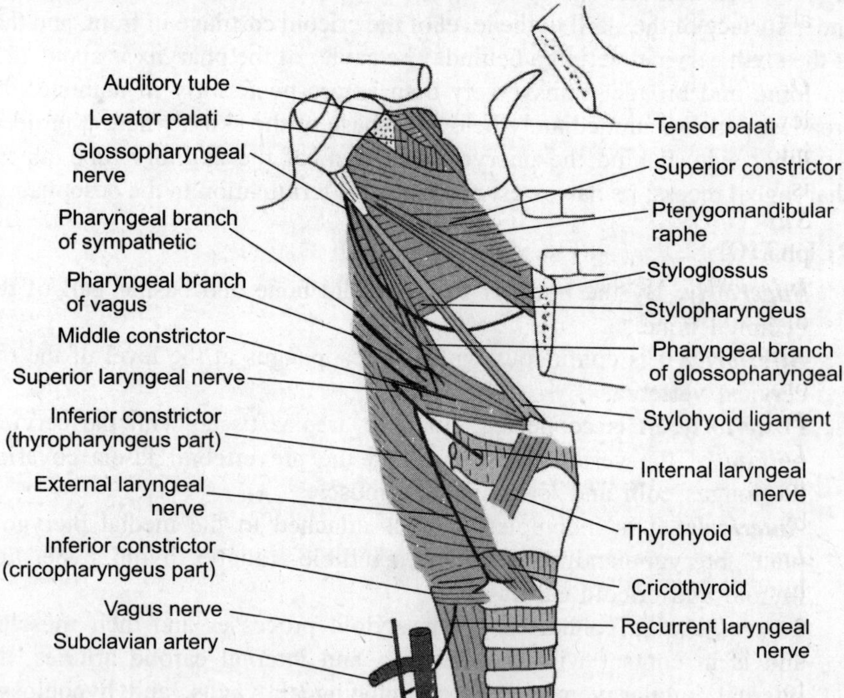

Fig. 10.1. The constrictors of pharynx.

RELATIONS

Anteriorly it communicates with the nasal cavities through the posterior nasal aperture.

Posteriorly Inferiorly it communicates with the oropharynx at the nasopharyngeal isthmus (it is an opening bounded by the lower border of the soft palate and the posterior wall of the pharynx).

Laterally

(a) the pharyngeal opening of the tube, at the level of the inferior nasal concha and about 1.2 cm. behind it.
(b) the tubal elevation bounds the tubal opening.
(c) the salpingopharyngeal fold is a vertical fold of mucous membrane running downwards from the posterior margin of the tubal elevation and gradually fades on the side wall of the pharynx. It is raised by the salpingopharyngeal muscle.
(d) as the levator palate enters the soft palate it raises a fold of mucous membrane below the tubal opening.
(e) there is a narrow vertical slit that leads into a flat pocket of mucous membrane called the pharyngeal recess. It extends sideways for half an inch or more between the auditory tube and prevertebral muscle, and above it lies the superior constrictor of pharynx.

Oropharynx Oral Part of Pharynx: reaches from the soft palate to the level of the hyoid bone. It opens anteriorly, through the isthmus faucium, into the mouth, while in its lateral wall, between the two palatine arches, is the palatine tonsil.
Superiorly: It communicates with the nasopharynx through the pharyngeal isthmus (nasopharyngeal isthmus).
Inferiorly: it opens into the laryngopharynx at the level of the border of the epiglottis.
Anteriorly: It communicates with the oral cavity through the oropharyngeal isthmus (isthmus of fauces)
Posteriorly: it is supported by the body of the axis vertebra.
Laterally: is the palatine tonsil which lies in the tonsillar fossa. This fossa is bounded anteriorly by the palatoglossal arch, and posteriorly by the superior, middle and inferior constrictors of pharynx.
Laryngopharynx Laryngeal Part of the Pharynx: reaches from the hyoid bone to the lower border of the cricoid cartilage, where it is continuous with the oesophagus. In front it presents the triangular entrance of the larynx, the base of which is directed forward and is formed by the epiglottis, while its lateral boundaries are constituted by the aryepiglottic folds. On either side of the laryngeal orifice is a recess, termed the sinus piriformis, which is bounded medially by the aryepiglottic fold, laterally by the thyroid cartilage and hypothyroid membrane.

RELATIONS

Anteriorly (a) the inlet of the larynx: and (b) the posterior surfaces of the cricoid and arytenoids cartilages.

Posteriorly is supported mainly by the 4th and 5th cervical vertebra and partly by the 3rd and 6th vertebrae. The posterior wall of the pharynx is formed by the superior, middle and inferior constrictor of pharynx.

Laterally there is a depression called the piriform fossa, one on each side of the inlet of the larynx. The fossa is bounded medially by the aryepiglottic fold, and laterally by the thyroid cartilage and the thyrohoid membrane. Beneath the mucosa of the fossa there lies the internal laryngeal nerve.

Inferior Constrictor Pharynx

Inferior constrictor pharynx is the thickest of the three constrictors.

Origin: from the side of the cricoid and thyroid cartilage. From the cricoid cartilage it arises in the interval between the cricothyroid in front, and the articular face for the inferior cornu of the thyroid cartilage behind. On the thyroid cartilage it arises from the oblique line on the side of the lamina, from the surface behind this nearly as far as the posterior border and from the inferior cornu. From these originis the fibres spread backward upward and medialward towards the median pharyngeal raphe.

Insertion: with the muscle of the opposite side into the fibrous raphe in the continuous with the circular fibres of the oesophagus; the rest ascend, increasing in obliquity, and overlap the middle constrictor of pharynx.

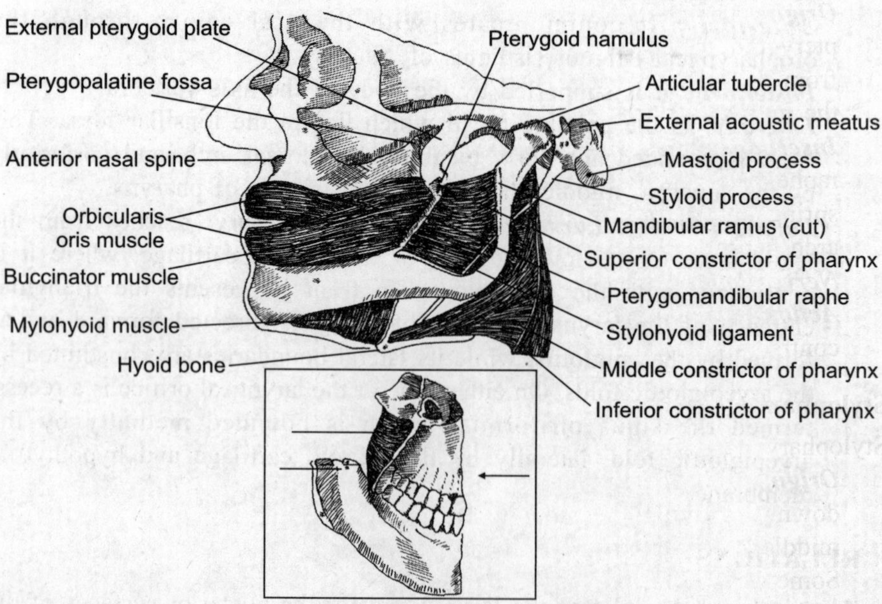

Fig. 10.2.

Nerve Supply: branches from the pharyngeal plexus and additional branches from the external laryngeal and recurrent nerves, and the stylopharyngeus by the glossopharyngeal nerve.

Action: by alternately contracting it forms a descending wave of contraction and help in pushing the bolus of food downwards.

Middle constrictor of pharynx

Middle constrictor of pharynx is a fan-shaped muscle, smaller than the preceding.

Origin: from the whole length of the upper border of the greater cornu of the hyoid bone, from the lesser cornu, and from the stylohyoid ligament. The fibres diverge from their the lower ones descend beneath the inferior constrictor, the middle fibres pass transversely, and the upper fibres ascend and overlap the superior constrictor.

Insertion: into the posterior median fibrous raphe, blending in the middle line with the muscle of the opposite side.

Nerve Supply: branches from the pharyngeal plexus

Action: by alternately contracting it forms a descending wave of contraction and help in pushing the bolus of food downwards.

Superior constrictor of pharynx

Superior constrictor of pharynx is a quadrilateral muscle, thinner and paler than the other two.

Origin: from the lower third of the posterior margin of the medial pterygoid plate and its Hamulus, from the pterygomandibular raphe, from the alveolar process of the mandible above the posterior end of the mylohyoid line, and by a few fibres from the side of the tongue.

Insertion: fibres curves backward and are inserted into the median raphe, being also prolonged by means of a aponeurosis to the pharyngeal spring on the basilar part of the occipital bone. The superior fibres arch beneath the levator veli palatine and the auditory tube.

Nerve supply: branches from the pharyngeal plexus

Action: by alternately contracting it forms a descending wave of contraction and help in pushing the bolus of food downwards.

Stylopharyngeus

Stylopharyngeus is a long, slender muscle, cylindrical above, flattended below.

Origin: from the medial side of the base of the styloid process, passes downward along the side of the pharynx between the superior and middle constrictors and spreads out beneath the mucous membrane. Some of its fibres are lost in the constrictor muscle, while others, joining with the pharyngopalatinus.

Insertion: into the posterior border of the thyroid cartil ge. The glossopharyngeal nerve runs on the lateral side of this mu le, and crosses over it to reach the tongue.

Nerve supply: Glossopharyngeal nerve.

Action: due to their attachment to the thyroid cartilage it helps in lifting up the larynx during swallowing.

Salpingopharyngeous

Origin: from the inferior part of the auditory tube near its orifice

Insertion: it passes downward and blends with the posterior fasciculus of the pharyngopalatinus.

Nerve supply: branches from the pharyngeal plexus

Action: opens the auditory tube during swallowing to equalize the pressure on either sides of the tympanic membrane.

Palatopharyngus

Origin: Posterior edge of the hard palate and the palatine aponeurosis

Insertion: Pharyngeal muscle and raphe. Posterolateral border of the thyroid cartilage.

Nerve supply: branches from the pharyngeal plexus

Action: opens the auditory tube during swallowing to equalize the pressure on either sides of the tympanic membrane.

Table 2. Muscles of Pharynx

Superior constrictor	Pteryogoid plate, pterygomandibular raphe, and mandible	Occipital bone and pharyngeal raphe	Constricts upper part of pharynx in deglutition	Pharyngeal branch of vagus n. (CN X)
Middle constrictor	Hyoid bone	Pharyngeal raphe	Constricts mid pharynx in deglutition	Pharyngeal branch of vagus n. (CN X)
Inferior constrictor	Thyroid cartilage	Pharyngeal raphe	Constricts upper part of pharynx in deglutition	Pharyngeal branch of vagus n. (CN X)
Palatopharyngeus	Palatine aponeurosis	Pharynx	Raises pharynx and larynx	Pharyngeal branch of vagus n. (CN X)
Salpingopharyngeus	Auditory tube	Pharynx	Raises pharynx and larynx	Pharyngeal branch of vagus n. (CN X)
Stylopharyngeus	Styloid process	Posterior border of thyroid cartilage and side wall of pharynx	Raises pharynx	Glosso-pharyngeal n. (CN IX)

Applied anatomy

1. Beneath the mucosa of the piriform fossa there lies the internal laryngeal nerve, removal of foreign bodies from the piriform fossa may damage the internal laryngeal nerve, leading to anesthesia in the supraglottic part of the larynx.

Hard Palate

It acts as a partition between the nasal and the oral cavities. Its anterior 2/3rd is formed by the palatine processes of maxillae, and its posterior 1/3rd by the horizontal plate of the palatine bones.

Anterolateral margins are continuous with the alveolar arches and gums; posterior margin gives attachment to the soft palate; superior forms the floor of the nose; inferior surface forms the roof of the oral cavity.

Nerve and vessels

Arteries greater palatine branch of the maxillary artey

Veins to the pterygold plexus of veins

Nerves greater and nasopalatine branches of the pterygopalatine ganglion (maxillary nerve)

Lymphatics drain mostly to the upper deep cervical nodes and partly to the retreopharyngeal nodes.

Soft Palate

It is a movable, muscular fold, suspended from the posterior border of the hard palate. It separates the nasopharynx from the oropharynse.

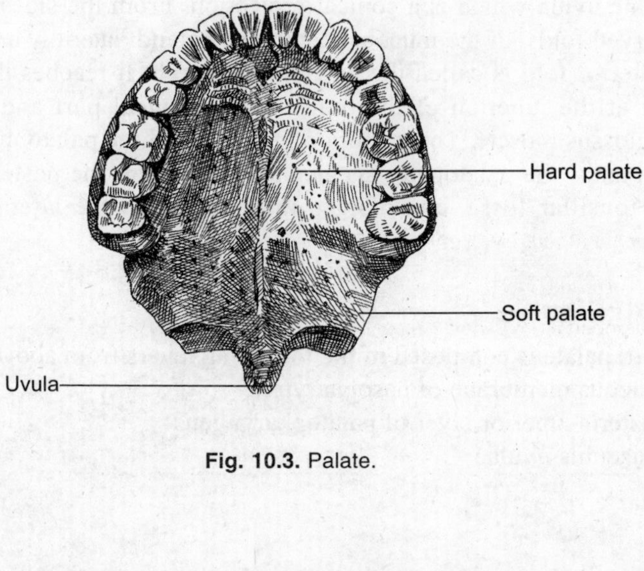

Fig. 10.3. Palate.

Surface

Anterior surface is concave and is marked by a raphe.

Posterior surface is convex, and is continuous superiorly with the floor of the nasal cavity.

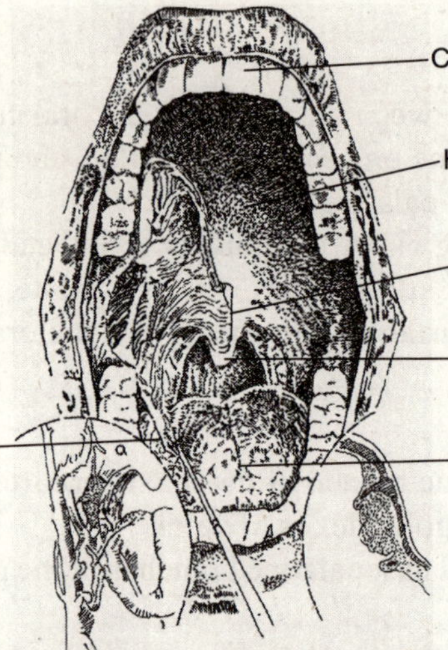

Fig. 10.4. Contents of the oral cavity.

Borders

Superior border is attached to the posterior border of the hard palate, blending on each side of the pharynx.

Inferior border is free and bounds the pharyngeal isthmus. From its middle hangs the uvula which is a conical projection. From the sides of the uvula, two curved folds of the mucous membrane extend laterally and downward. The anterior fold is called the palatoglossal arch. It reaches the side of the tongue at the junction of the oral and pharyngeal part and contains the palatoglossus muscle. The posterior fold is called the palatopharyngeal arch and contains the palatopharyngeus muscle. It forms the posterior boundary of the tonsillar fossa, and merges inferiorly with the lateral wall of the pharynx.

Structure

The soft palate is composed of the following layers from above downwards:

1. Mucous membrane of nasopharynx
2. Postero-superior layer of palatopharyngeus
3. Musculus uvulae

4. Levator palate muscle
5. Antero-inferior layer of palatopharyngeus
6. Tendon of tensor palati
7. Palatoglossus muscle
8. Buccal mucous membrane with salivary glands and lymph tissue.

Arterial supply

1. The greater palatine branch of the maxillary artey.
2. The ascending palatine branch of the facial artery
3. The palatine branch of the ascending pharyngeal artery

Venous drainage: They pass to the pterygoid and tonsillar plescuses of the veins

Lymphatic drainage: It drains into the upper deep cervical and retropharyngeal lymph nodes.

Applied anatomy

1. Paralysis of the soft palate in case of a lesion of the vagus nerve causes regurgitation of food and liquid from the nose and a nasal tinge in the voice.
2. Air travellers are encouraged to swallow by the distribution of toffees or gums by the air hostess so that the auditory tube can be kept open during take off and landing in order to equalize the pressure on either sides of the tympanic membrane.
3. Cleft palate, which is a developmental defect, results from the non-fusion of shelf-like palatine processes of the maxillary protuberance.

Muscles

Tensor palati

Origin: it originates from the lateral side of the auditory tube and the adjoining part of the base of the greater wing and scaphoid fossa of the sphenoid bone.

Insertion: the muscle descends and converges to form a tendon which winds around the pterygoid hamulus, then it passes through the origin of the buccinator muscle and then it flattens out to form the palatine aponeurosis. Aponeurosis is attached to the posterior border of the hard palate and the inferior surface of the hard palate behind the palatine crest.

Nerve supply: By a branch from the trunk of the mandibular nerve which passes through the otic ganglion without relaying in it.

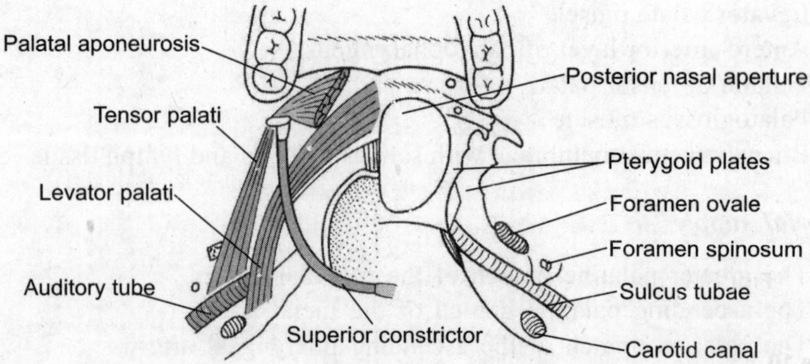

Fig. 10.5. Two muscles (tensor palati and levator palati) enter the soft palate from above.

Action: it tenses the soft palate mainly the anterior part and opens the auditory tube to equalize the air pressure on either side of the tympanic membrane.

Levator Palati

Origin: the inferior aspect of the auditory tube and the adjoining part of the inferior surface of the petrous part of the temporal bone.
Insertion: the muscle enters the pharynx by passing over the upper concave margin of the superior constrictor of pharynx and then it runs downwards and medially and spreads out in the soft palate. It is inserted in the upper surface of the palatine aponeurosis.
Nerve supply: cranial part of the accessory nerve through the pharyngeal plexus
Action: it elevates the soft palate and closes the nasopharyngeal isthmus. It also opens the auditory tube to equalise the air pressure on either side of the tympanic membrane.

Musculus Uvulae

Origin: Posterior edge of the hard palate
Insertion: Mucous membrane of uvulae
Nerve supply: Cranial part of the accessory nerve through the pharyngeal plxus
Action: Pulls up the uvulae

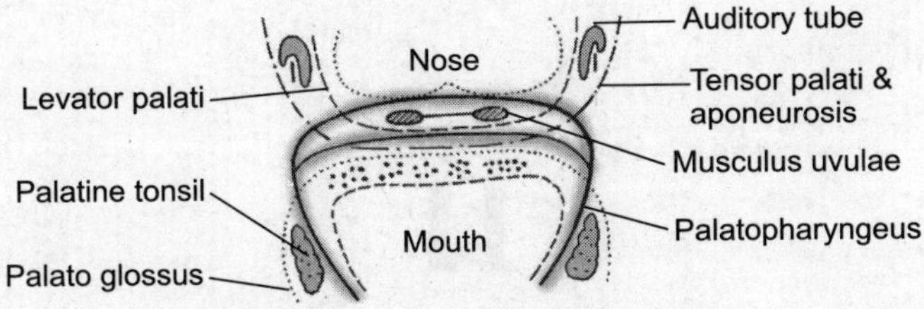

Fig. 10.6. Scheme showing the muscular composition of the soft palate.

Table 10.1. Muscles of the Soft Palate.

Muscle	Origin	Insertion	Action	Innervation
Palatine musculature				
Tensor veli palatine	Lateral surface of auditory auditory tube	Velum via hamulus	Tenses velum	Mandibular n. (CN V3)
Levator veli palatine	Temporal bone and medial surface of auditory tube	Velum	Raises velum	Pharyngeal branch of vagus n. (CN X)
Palatoglossus	Palatine aponeurosis	Tongue	Raises tongue	Pharyngeal branch of vagus n. (CN X)
Palatopharyngeus	Palatine aponeurosis	1. Posterior of hard palate 2. Posterior border of thyroid cartilage	Raises larynx	Pharyngeal branch of vagus n. (CN X)

11
Larynx

The larynx comprises a series of sphincters placed at the upper part of the air passage. It is located between the trachea and the root of the tongue, at the upper and forepart of the neck. Its vertical extent corresponds to the fourth, fifth, and sixth cervical vertebrae, but it is placed somewhat higher in the female and also during childhood. The average measurements of the adult larynx are as follows:

	In males	In females
Length	44 mm	36 mm
Transverse diameter	43 mm	41 mm
Antero-posterior diameter	36 mm	26 mm
Circumference	136 mm	112 mm

Until puberty the larynx of the male differs little in size from that of the female. In the female its increase after puberty is only slight; in the male it undergoes considerable prominent in the midline of the neck, while the length of the rima glottides is nearly doubled.

There are 3 paired and 3 unpaired cartilages of larynx.

The paired cartilages are:

1. Arytenoid 2
2. Corniculate 2
3. Cuneiform 2

The unpaired carilages are

1. Thyroid 1
2. Cricoid 1
3. Epiglottis 1

Total number of cartilages is 9

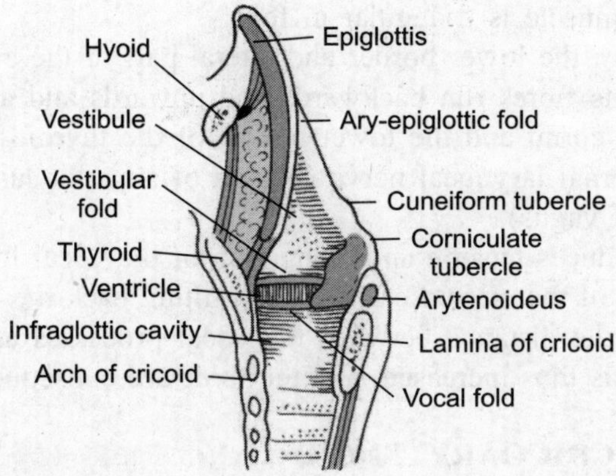

Fig. 11.1. Interior of larynx in sagittal section showing its three parts.

MUSCLES

The intrinsic muscles are:

1. Cricothyroid
2. Posterior cricoary tenoid
3. Thyroarytenoid
4. Lateral cricoarytenoid
5. Transverse arytenoid
6. Oblique arytenoid
7. Aryepiglotticus
8. Thyroepiglotticus
9. Vocalis

Thus the total number of muscles is also 9.

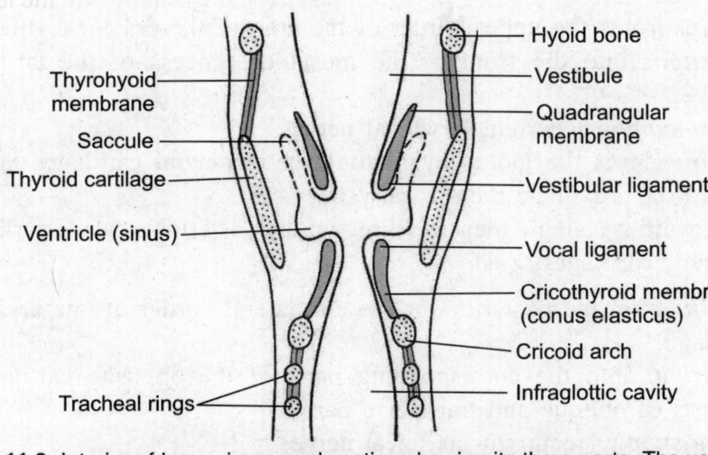

Fig. 11.2. Interior of larynx in coronal section showing its three parts. The vestibule is like a truncated inverted hollow cone while the infraglottic part is like a truncated erect hollow cone. Ventricle is the outward bulge between the two.

Cricothyroid: muscle is triangular in form

Origin: from the lower border and lateral part of the cricoid cartilage;

Insertion: its fibres run backwards and upwards and are inserted into the inferior cornu and the lower border of the thyroid cartilage.

Nerve: external laryngeal nerve (branch of superior laryngeal nerve—a branch of vagus)

Action: produces tension and elongation of the vocal folds by drawing up the arch of the cricoid cartilage and tilting back the upper border of its lamina; the distance between the vocal processes and the angle of the thyroid is thus increased, and the folds are consequently elongated.

POSTERIOR CRICOARYTENOID

Origin: forms the broad depression on the corresponding half of the posterior surface of the lamina of the cricoid cartilage.

Insertion: into the back of the muscular process of the arytenoids cartilage. The uppermost fibres are nearly horizontal, the middle oblique, and the lowest are almost vertical.

Nerve supply: recurrent laryngeal nerve (branch of vagus).

Action: separates the vocal folds, and, consequently, opens the glottis, by rotating the arytenoid cartilages outward around a vertical axis passing through the cricoarytenoid joins so that their vocal processes and the vocal folds attached to them become widely separated. Thus, it is the safety muscle of larynx, and safeguards from asphyxiation (details given under applied anatomy).

Lateral cricoarytenoid is smaller than the preceding, and of an oblong form.

Origin: froms the upper border of the arch of the cricoid cartilage.

Insertion: into the front of the muscular process of the arytenoid carilage.

Nerve supply: recurrent laryngeal nerve.

Action: closes the glottis by rotating the arytenoid cartilages inward, so as to approximate their vocal processes.

Arytenoid is a single muscle, filling up the posterior concave surface of the arytenoid cartilages.

Origin: from the posterior surface and lateral border of one arytenoid cartilage.

Insertion: into the corresponding parts of the opposite cartilage. It consists of oblique and transverse parts.

Nerve supply: recurrent laryngeal nerve.

Action: approximates the arytenoid cartilages, and thus closes the opening of the glottis, especially at its back part.

Thyroarytenoid is a broad, thin, muscle which lies parallel with and lateral to the vocal fold, and supports the wall of the ventricle and its appendix

Origin: in front from the lower half of the angle of the thyroid cartilage, and from the middle cricothyroid ligament. Its fibres pass backward and lateralward

Insertion: into the base and anterior surface of the arytenoid cartilage.

Nerve supply: recurrent laryngeal nerve

Action: the main use is to draw the arytenoids cartilages forward towards the thyroid, and thus shortens and relaxes the vocal folds.

Arterial supply of the larynx

1. The superior laryngeal artery, a branch of the superior thyroid artery supplies upto the vocal folds
2. The inferior laryngeal artery, a branch of the inferior thyroid artery supplies below the vocal folds

Table 11.1. Intrinsic muscles of the larynx

Muscle	Origin	Insertion	Action	Innervation
Cricothyroid	Cricoid cartilage anteriorly	Thyroid cartilage laterally	Stretches and tenses vocal cords	Superior (external) laryngeal branch of vagus n. (CN X)
Posterior cricoarytenoid	Cricoid cartilage posteriorly	Arytenoid cartilage	Abducts vocal cords	Inferior (recurrent) laryngeal branch of vagus nerve (CN X)
Lateral cricoarytenoid	Arytenoid cartilage	Arytenoid cartilage	Abducts vocal cords (safety muscle)	Inferior (recurrent) laryngeal branch of vagus nerve (CN X)
Thyroarytenoid (vocalis)	Thyroid cartilage anteriorly	Arytenoid cartilage	Abducts and tenses vocal cords	Inferior (recurrent) laryngeal branch of vagus nerve (CN X)

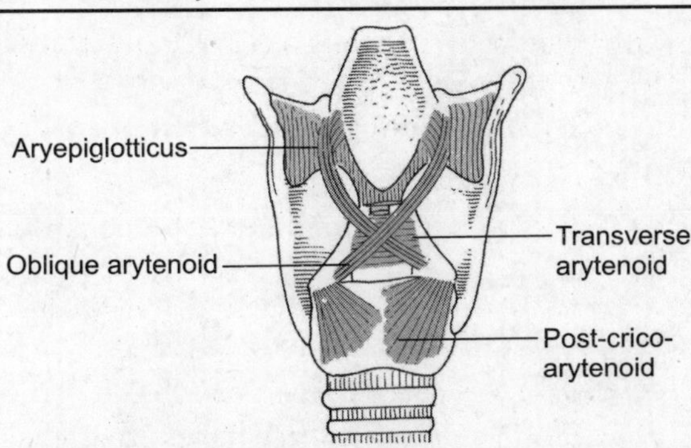

Fig. 11.3. The intrinsic muscles of larynx in posterior view.

Applied anatomy

1. ***Safety muscle*** the posterior cricoarytenoid muscle is called the safety muscle because all the intrinsic muscles are adductors of the vocal cords except posterior cricoarytenoid which are abductors. The space between two vocal cords called rima glottis is the narrowest space in the lumen of larynx. The patency of glottis is essential for the entry and exit of air, the two vital components of respiration. The glottis is narrowed by adduction of vocal cords and widening by the abduction.

Since the integrity of posterior cricoarytenoid muscle saves the life of a person, because if they are paralysed, the action of the abductor muscles will be unopposed, and a person may die due to lack of air. Hence the posterior cricoarytenoid is known as the safety muscle of the larynx.

2. ***Heimlich manoeuver*** if a foreign body gets lodged in the larynx (rima glottides), it causes laryngeal obstruction (choking). Because the lungs up through the trachea to expel the food or other foreign body and clear the obstruction. Since the larynx is the narrowest part of the respiratory passage, foreign bodies are usually lodged here.
3. ***Laryngitis*** infection and inflammation of the larynx. It is caused by hoarsenss of voice and temporary loss of voice.
4. ***Laryngoscopy*** the various structures of the larynx can be seen directly by means of a laryngoscope. The various structure seen are the base of the tongue, the valleculae, aryepiglottic folds, piriform fossae, vestibular folds, epiglottis, vocal cords. It is of great clinical importance.
5. ***Paralysis*** when both recurrent laryngeal nerves are damaged the vocal chords lie in between the position of abduction and abduction phonation (voice production) is completely lost. Breathing also becomes difficult through the partially opened glottis. When only one recurrent laryngeal nerve is paralysed the opposite nerve compensates for it and phonation is possible.

12

Parasympathetic Ganglia

CILIARY GANGLION

Location: near the apex of the orbit, between the optic nerve and lateral rectus.

Size: is of a pin-head

Roots:

1. Parasympathetic root from the inferior branch of the oculomotor nerve. Preganglionic fibres are relayed in the ciliary ganglion and supply the sphincter pupillae and ciliary muscle.
2. Sensory fibres from the eyeball to the maxillary nerve which is a branch of the opthalmic nerve.
3 Sympathetic postganglionic fibres coming from the superior cervical ganglion to supply the dilator muscles of the pupil and superior and inferior tarsal muscles.

Branches: Fifteen to twenty short ciliary nerves piercing the back of the eyeball with the optic nerve.

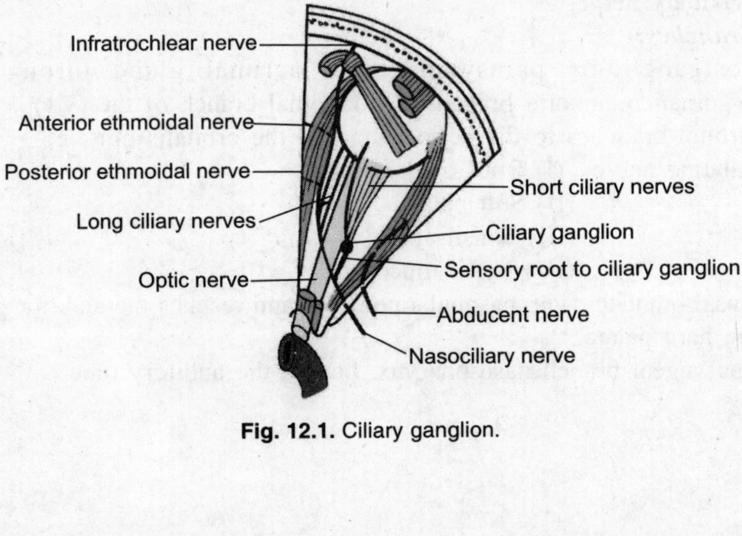

Fig. 12.1. Ciliary ganglion.

Pterygopalatine or Meckel's ganglion

This ganglion is connected with the maxillary division of the Vth nerve

Location: in the upper part of the pterygopalatine fossa and is the size of the head of a small tack.

Roots: Motor root (parasympathetic root). The fibres leave the brain stem in nervus intermedius, join the VIIth nerve, and leave facial (geniculate) ganglion as the greater superficial petrosal nerve.

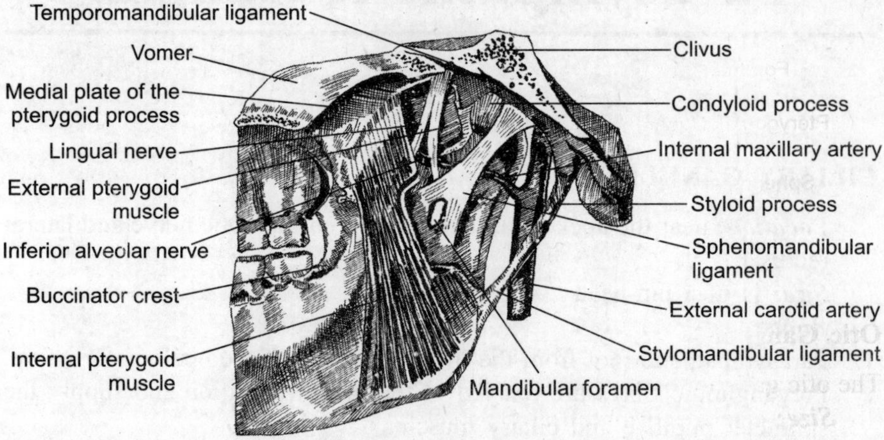

Fig. 12.2. Pterygo palatine region.

Sympathetic root: The cell bodies are in the superior cervical ganglion, pass to the internal carotid plexus. Deep petrosal nerve, joins the greater superficial petrosal nerve to form the nerve of the pterygoid canal.

Sensory root: cell bodies in the trigeminal ganglion. Comes from the maxillary nerve.

Branches:

1. Postganglionic parasympathetic lacrimal gland through the zygomaticotemporal branch (V2) lacrimal branch of the (V1)
2. Orbital branches to the periosteum and the orbitalis muscle.
3. Palatine nerves (I) Roof of the mouth
   (II) Soft palate
   (III) Tonsil and
   (IV) Nasal mucosa
4. Nasal branches, via, nasopalatine nerve and reaches the anterior part of the hard palate.
5. Pharyngeal branch naso-pharynx, behind the auditory tube.

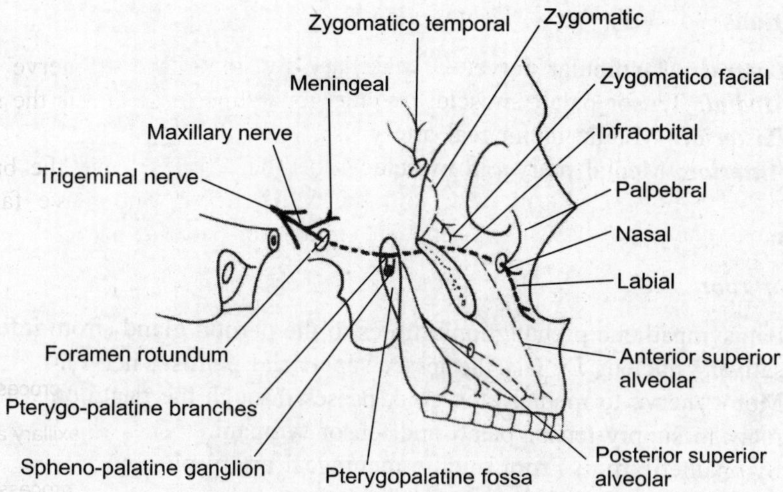

Fig. 12.3. Pterygo palatine ganglion.

Otic Ganglion

The otic ganglion is connected to the mandibular (V3)

Size: size of a pinhead (2×1mm).

Location: It is situated medial to the trunk of the mandibular nerve (V3) at the base of the skull just outside the foramen ovale.

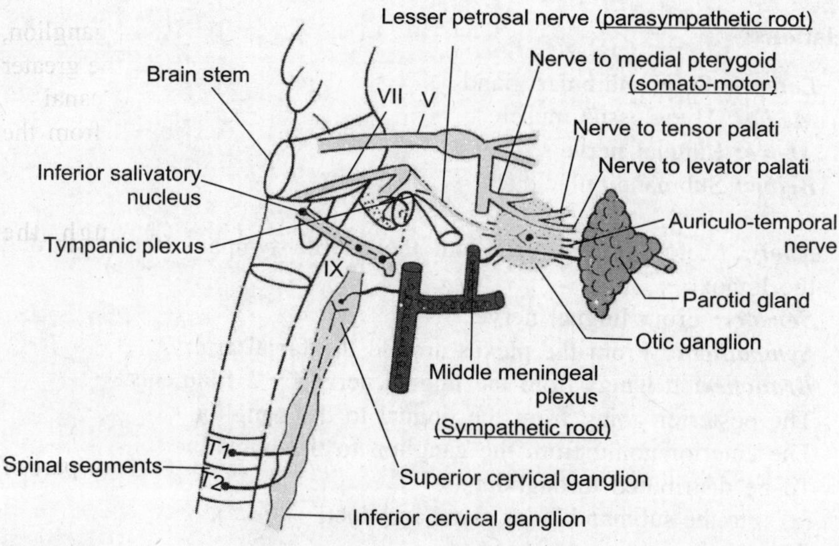

Fig. 12.4. Otic ganglion.

Relations

Lateral: Mandibular nerve.
Medial: Tensor palate muscle
Posterior: Middle meningeal artery
Anterior: Medial pterygoid muscle

Roots

Motor root

1. Parasympathetic preganglionic fibres to the parotid gland (from inferior salivary nucleus IX CN the lesser superficial petrosal nerve).
2. Motor: nerve to medial pterygoid, passes through the ganglion without relay to supply tensor palati and tensor tympani.
3. Sympathetic root: From middle meningeal artery plexus
4. Sensory: Fine twigs from the auriculotemporal nerve.

Branches: with the exception of the 2 motor branches supplying the 2 tensor muscles, all branches are distributed to the parotid gland. Travelling with the auriculotemporal nerve.

Submandibular or Langley's ganglion

Location: situated on the outer surface of the hyoglossus muscle suspended from the lingual nerve.
Size: pin-head

Relations

Lateral: Submandibular gland
Medial: Hyoglossus muscle
Above: Lingual nerve
Below: Submandibular duct

Roots: Motor (secretory): From the chorda tympani (facial) through the lingual
Sensory: From lingual nerve
Sympathetic: From the plexus around the facial artery.
Branches: It hangs from the lingual nerve by 2 filaments,
The posterior going from the lingual to the ganglion.
The anterior going from the ganglion to the lingual
To be distributed throughout.
(a) to the submandibular gland and duct;
(b) to the sublingual gland

(c) to the mucous membrane of the mouth and tongue (through the lingual nerve)

Pathway for taste

1. Taste sensation in the anterior 2/3rd of the tongue passes via the lingual nerve to the chorda tympani. Thence to the facial nerve in the canal for the facial nerve. And so to the geniculate ganglion. Whence the impulses go in the nervus intermedius (VII CN) to the pons.
2. From posterior 1/3rd of the tongue taste sensation passes via the IXth CN to brain stem. Temporary loss of taste over the anterior 2/3rd of the tongue may follow removal of the trigeminal ganglion. This is due to the swelling of the axons of the lingual nerve consequent on their degeneration.

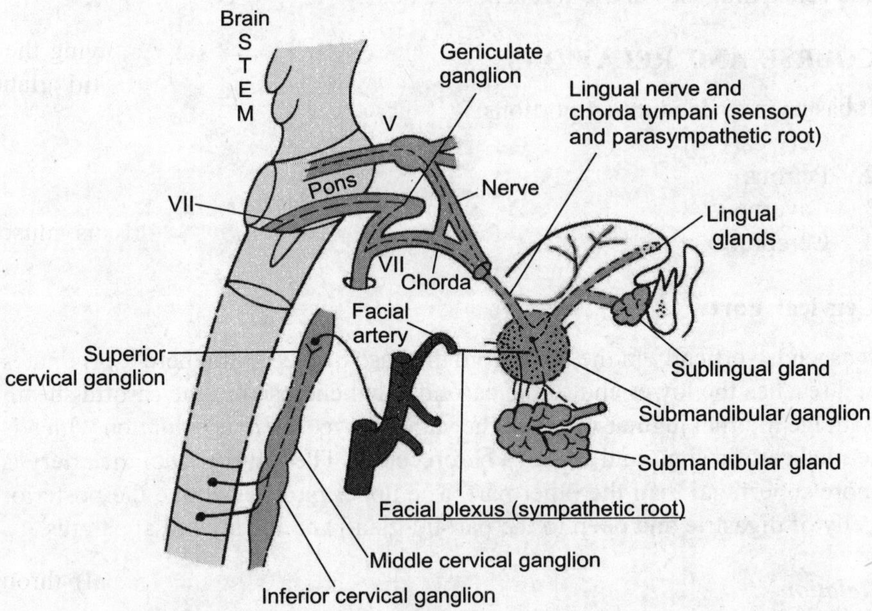

Fig. 12.5. Submandibular ganglion–roots and branches.

13
Arteries of Head and Neck

INTERNAL CAROTID ARTERY

Internal carotid artery is one of the 2 terminal branches of the common carotid artery and supplies the anterior part of the brain, the eye and its appendages, and sends branches to the forehead and nose.

COURSE AND RELATIONS

It has been divided into 4 portions:

1. Cervical
2. Petrous
3. Cavernous
4. Cerebral

Cervical Part

It ascends vertically in the neck from the base of the skull where it originates and reaches the lower end of the carotid canal enclosed in the carotid sheath with the internal jugular vein and the vagus nerve. There is a dilation which is termed carotid sinus and acts as a baroreceptor. The lower part of the artery is more superficial than the other part. The upper part lies above the posterior belly of digastric and deep to the parotid gland and the styloid apparatus.

Relation

Behind: with the longus capitis, the superior cervical ganglion of the sympathetic trunk, and the superior laryngeal nerve.

Laterally: with the internal jugular vein and vagus nerve, the nerve lying on a plane posterior to the artery.

Medially: with the pharynx, superior laryngeal nerve, and ascending pharyngeal artery.

Inferiorly: the glossopharyngeal, vagus, accessory and hypoglossal nerves lie between the artery and the internal jugular vein.

Branches: The cervical portion of the internal carotid gives off no branches.

Petrous part

Course: the artery enters the canal in the petrous portion of the temporal bone, it ascends, then curves forward and medialward and again ascends as it leaves the canal to enter the cavity of the skull between the lingual and petrosal process of the sphenoid.

Relations: the artery lies in front of the cochlea and tympanic cavity; it is separated by cribriform palate. Further forward it is separated from the trigeminal ganglion by a thin plate of bone, which forms the floor of the fossa for the ganglion and the roof of the horizontal portion of the canal.The artery is separated from the bony wall of the carotid canal by a prolongation of dura mater, and is surrounded by a number of small veins and by filaments of the carotid plexus, derived from the ascending branch of the superior cervical ganglion of the sympathetic trunk.

Cavernous Part

Cavernous part the artery is situated between the layers of the dura mater forming the cavernous sinus, and are covered by the lining membrane of the sinus. At first it ascends toward the posterior clinoid process, then passes forward by the side of the body of the sphenoid bone, and again curves upward on the medial side of the anterior clinoid process, and perforates the dura mater forming the roof of the sinus. This portion of the artery is surrounded by filaments of the sympathetic nerve, and on its lateral side is the abducent nerve.

Branches of the cavernous part are:

1. Cavernous
2. Hypophyseal
3. Semilunar
4. Anterior meningeal
5. Opthalmic

Cerebral part having perforated the dura mater on the medial side of the anterior clinoid process, the internal carotid artery passes between the optic and oculomotor nerves to the medial side of the lateral cerebral fissure, where it gives off its terminal or cerebral branches.

Branches of the cerebral part:

1. Anterior cerebral
2. Middle cerebral
3. Posterior communicating
4. Choroidal

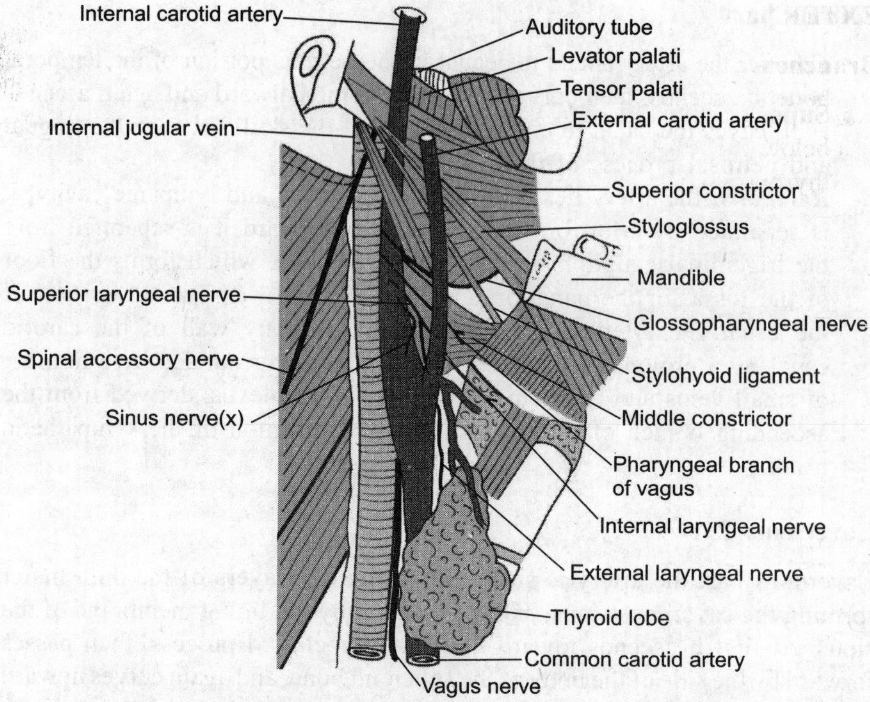

Fig. 13.1. Medial relations of internal and external carotid arteries.

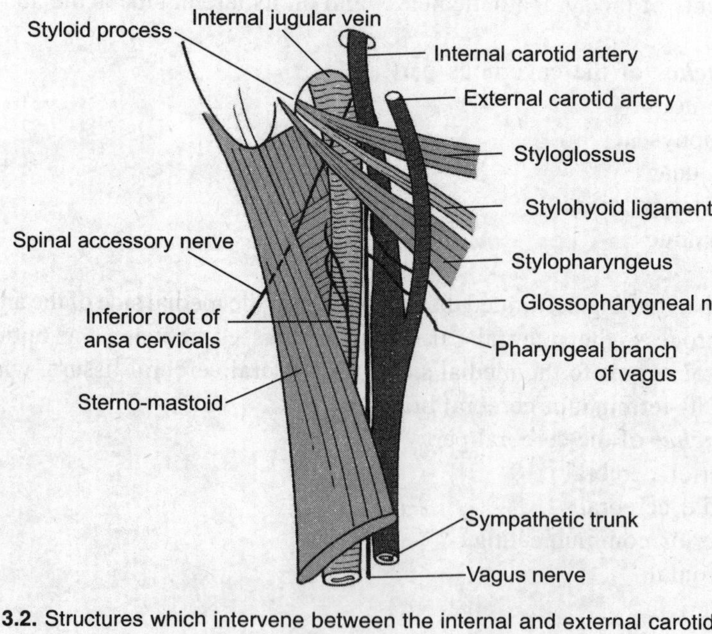

Fig. 13.2. Structures which intervene between the internal and external carotid arteries.

EXTERNAL CAROTID ARTERY

Branches

1. **Superior thyroid artery** arises from the external carotid artery just below the level of the greater cornu of the hyoid bone and ends in the thyroid gland.
   - ***Hyoid Branch:*** is small and runs along the lower border of the hyoid bone beneath the thyrohyoid and anastomoses with the vessel of the opposite side.
   - ***sternocleidomastoid Branch:*** runs downward and lateralward across the sheath of the common carotid artery, and supplies the Sternocleidomastoid and neighboring muscles and integument; it frequently arises as a separate branch from the external carotid.
   - ***Superior Laryngeal Artery:*** larger than either of the preceding, accompanies the internal laryngeal branch of the superior laryngeal nerve, beneath the Thyrohyoid; it pierces the thyrohyoid membrane, and supplies the muscles, mucous membrane, and glands of the larynx, anastomosing with the branch from the opposite side.
   - ***Cricothyroid Branch:*** is small and runs transversely across the cricothyroid membrane, communicating with the artery of the opposite side.
2. **Lingual artery** arises from the external carotid between the superior thyroid and facial artery; it first runs obliquely upward and medialward to the greater cornu of the hyoid bone; it then curves downward and forward, forming a loop which is crossed by the hypoglossal nerve, and passing beneath the digastric and stylohyoid it runs horizontally forward, beneath the hyoglossus, and finally, ascending almost perpendicularly to the tongue, turns forward on its lower surface as far as the tip.
   - ***Hyoid Branch:*** runs along the upper border of the hyoid bone, supplying the muscles attached to it and anastomosing with its fellow of the opposite side.
   - ***Arteriæ Dorsales Linguii:*** consist usually of two or three small branches which arise beneath the hyoglossus; they ascend to the back part of the dorsum of the tongue, and supply the mucous membrane in this situation, the glossopalatine arch, the tonsil, soft palate, and epiglottis; anastomosing with the vessels of the opposite side.
   - ***Sublingual Artery:*** arises at the anterior margin of the hyoglossus, and runs forward between the genioglossus and mylohyoid to the sublingual gland. It supplies the gland and gives branches to the mylohyoid and neighboring muscles, and to the mucous membrane

of the mouth and gums. One branch runs behind the alveolar process of the mandible in the substance of the gum to anastomose with a similar artery from the other side; another pierces the mylohyoid and anastomoses with the submental branch of the external maxillary artery.

- ***Arteria profunda linguii:*** also called ranine artery or the deep lingual artery is the terminal portion of the lingual artery; it pursues a tortuous course and runs along the under surface of the tongue, above the mucous membrane; it lies on the lateral side of the genioglossus, accompanied by the lingual nerve. At the tip of the tongue, it is said to anastomose with the artery of the opposite side. In the mouth, these vessels are placed one on either side of the lingual frenulum.

3. **Facial artery** also sometimes referred as the external maxillary artery it arises in the carotid triangle just above the lingual artery and, is covered by the ramus of the mandible, it passes obliquely up beneath the digastric and stylohyoid, over which it arches to enter a groove on the posterior surface of the submandibular gland. It then curves upward over the body of the mandible at the antero-inferior angle of the masseter; passes forward and upward across the cheek to the angle of the mouth, then ascends along the side of the nose, and ends at the medial commissure of the eye, under the name of the angular artery. This vessel, both in the neck and on the face, is remarkably tortuous: in the former situation, to accommodate itself to the movements of the pharynx in deglutition; and in the latter, to the movements of the mandible, lips, and cheeks.

- ***Ascending Palatine Artery:*** arises close to the origin of the external maxillary artery and passes up between the styloglossus and stytopharyngeus to the side of the pharynx, along which it is continued between the superior constrictor of pharynx and the pterygoid to near the base of the skull. It divides near the levator veli palatini into two branches: one follows the course of this muscle, and, winding over the upper border of the superior constrictor of pharynx, supplies the soft palate and the palatine glands, anastomosing with the artery of the opposite side and with the descending palatine branch of the internal maxillary artery; the other pierces the superior constrictor of pharynx and supplies the palatine tonsil and auditory tube, anastomosing with the tonsillar and ascending pharyngeal arteries.
- ***Tonsillar Branch:*** ascends between the pterygoid and styloglossus, and then along the side of the pharynx, perforating the superior constrictor of pharynx, to ramify in the substance of the palatine tonsil and root of the tongue.

- **Glandular Branches:** consist of three or four large vessels, which supply the submandibular gland, some being prolonged to the neighboring muscles, lymph glands, and integument.
- **Submental Artery:** the largest of the cervical branches, is given off from the facial artery just as that vessel quits the submandibular gland: it runs forward upon the mylohyoid, just below the body of the mandible, and beneath the digastric. It supplies the surrounding muscles, and anastomoses with the sublingual artery and with the mylohyoid branch of the inferior alveolar; at the symphysis menti it turns upward over the border of the mandible and divides into a superficial and a deep branch.
- **Inferior Labial Artery:** arises near the angle of the mouth; it passes upward and forward beneath the triangularis and, penetrating the orbicularis oris, runs in a tortuous course along the edge of the lower lip between this muscle and the mucous membrane. It supplies the labial glands, the mucous membrane, and the muscles of the lower lip; and anastomoses with the artery of the opposite side, and with the mental branch of the inferior alveolar artery.
- **Superior Labial Artery:** is larger and more tortuous than the inferior. It follows a similar course along the edge of the upper lip, lying between the mucous membrane and the orbicularis oris, and anastomoses with the artery of the opposite side. It supplies the upper lip, and gives off in its course two or three vessels which ascend to the nose; a *septal branch* ramifies on the nasal septum as far as the point of the nose, and an *alar branch* supplies the ala of the nose.
- **Lateral Nasal:** branch derive from the external maxillary as that vessel ascends along the side of the nose. It supplies the ala and dorsum of the nose, anastomosing with its fellow, with the septal and alar branches, with the dorsal nasal branch of the ophthalmic, and with the infraorbital branch of the internal maxillary.
- **Angular Artery:** is the terminal part of the external maxillary; it ascends to the medial angle of the orbit, imbedded in the fibres of the angular head of the quadratus labii superioris, and accompanied by the angular vein. On the cheek it distributes branches which anastomose with the infraorbital; after supplying the lacrimal sac and orbicularis oculi, it ends by anastomosing with the dorsal nasal branch of the ophthalmic artery.
- **Muscular Branches:** in the neck are distributed to the pterygoid and stylohyoid, and on the face to the masseter and buccinator. The anastomoses of the external maxillary artery are very numerous, not only with the vessel of the opposite side, but, *in the neck,* with the sublingual branch of the lingual, with the ascending pharyngeal,

and by its ascending palatine and tonsillar branches with the palatine branch of the internal maxillary; *on the face,* with the mental branch of the inferior alveolar as it emerges from the mental foramen, with the transverse facial branch of the superficial temporal, with the infraorbital branch of the internal maxillary, and with the dorsal nasal branch of the ophthalmic.

4. **Occipital artery** arises from the posterior part of the external carotid, opposite the facial artery, near the lower margin of the posterior belly of the digastric, and ends in the posterior part of the scalp.
   - ***Muscular Branches:*** supply the digastric, stylohyoid, splenius, and longissimus capitis.
   - ***Sternocleidomastoid Artery:*** generally arises from the occipital close to its commencement, but sometimes springs directly from the external carotid. It passes downward and backward over the hypoglossal nerve, and enters the substance of the muscle, in company with the accessory nerve.
   - ***Auricular Branch:*** supplies the back of the concha and frequently gives off a branch, which enters the skull through the mastoid foramen and supplies the dura mater, the diploë, and the mastoid cells; this latter branch sometimes arises from the occipital artery, and is then known as the *mastoid branch.*
   - ***Meningeal Branch:*** ascends with the internal jugular vein, and enters the skull through the jugular foramen and condyloid canal, to supply the dura mater in the posterior fossa.
   - ***Descending Branch:*** the largest branch of the occipital, descends on the back of the neck, and divides into a superficial and deep portion. The superficial portion runs beneath the splenius, giving off branches which pierce that muscle to supply the trapezius and anastomose with the ascending branch of the transverse cervical: the deep portion runs down between the semispinales capitis and colli, and anastomoses with the vertebral and with the arteria profunda cervicalis, a branch of the costocervical trunk. The anastomosis between these vessels assists in establishing the collateral circulation after ligature of the common carotid or subclavian artery.

5. **Posterior auricular artery** is small and arises from the external carotid, above the digastric and stylohyoid, opposite the apex of the styloid process. It ascends, undercover of the parotid gland, on the styloid process of the temporal bone, to the groove between the cartilage of the ear and the mastoid process, immediately above which it divides into its auricular and occipital branches.
   - ***Stylomastoid Artery:*** enters the stylomastoid foramen and supplies the tympanic cavity, the tympanic antrum and mastoid cells, and

the semicircular canals. In the young subject a branch from this vessel forms, with the anterior tympanic artery from the internal maxillary, a vascular circle, which surrounds the tympanic membrane, and from which delicate vessels ramify on that membrane. It anastomoses with the superficial petrosal branch of the middle meningeal artery by a twig which enters the hiatus canalis facialis.

- ***Auricular Branch:*** ascends behind the ear, beneath the auricularis posterior, and is distributed to the back of the auricula, upon which it ramifies minutely, some branches curving around the margin of the cartilage, others perforating it, to supply the anterior surface. It anastomoses with the parietal and anterior auricular branches of the superficial temporal.
- ***Occipital Branch:*** passes backward, over the sternocleidomastoid, to the scalp above and behind the ear. It supplies the occipitalis and the scalp in this situation and anastomoses with the occipital artery.

6. **Ascending pharyngeal artery,** the smallest branch of the external carotid, is a long, slender vessel, deeply seated in the neck, beneath the other branches of the external carotid and under the stylopharyngeus. It arises from the back part of the external carotid, near the commencement of that vessel, and ascends vertically between the internal carotid and the side of the pharynx, to the undersurface of the base of the skull, lying on the longus capitis.
   - ***Pharyngeal Branches:*** are three or four in number. Two of these descend to supply the middle and inferior constrictor of pharynx and the stylopharyngeus, ramifying in their substance and in the mucous membrane lining them.
   - ***Palatine Branch:*** varies in size, and may take the place of the ascending palatine branch of the facial artery, when that vessel is small. It passes inward upon the superior constrictor of pharynx sends ramifications to the soft palate and tonsil, and supplies a branch to the auditory tube.
   - ***Prevertebral Branches:*** are numerous small vessels, which supply the longi capitis and colli, the sympathetic trunk, the hypoglossal and vagus nerves, and the lymph glands; they anastomose with the ascending cervical artery.
   - ***Inferior Tympanic Artery:*** is a small branch which passes through a minute foramen in the petrous portion of the temporal bone, in company with the tympanic branch of the glossopharyngeal nerve, to supply the medial wall of the tympanic cavity and anastomose with the other tympanic arteries.
   - ***Meningeal Branches:*** are several small vessels, which supply the

dura mater. One, the *posterior meningeal,* enters the cranium through the jugular foramen; a second passes through the foramen lacerum; and occasionally a third through the canal for the hypoglossal nerve.

7. **Superficial temporal artery** the smaller of the two terminal branches of the external carotid, appears, from its direction, to be the continuation of that vessel. It begins in the substance of the parotid gland, behind the neck of the mandible, and crosses over the posterior root of the zygomatic process of the temporal bone; about 5 cm above this process it divides into two branches, a frontal and a parietal.
   - ***Transverse Facial Artery:*** is givien off from the superficial temporal before that vessel quits the parotid gland; running forward through the substance of the gland, it passes transversely across the side of the face, between the parotid duct and the lower border of the zygomatic arch, and divides into numerous branches, which supply the parotid gland and duct, the masseter, and the integument, and anastomose with the external maxillary, masseteric, buccinator, and infraorbital arteries. This vessel rests on the masseter, and is accompanied by one or two branches of the facial nerve.
   - ***Middle Temporal Artery:*** arises immediately above the zygomatic arch, and, perforating the temporal fascia, gives branches to the temporalis, anastomosing with the deep temporal branches of the internal maxillary. It occasionally gives off a zygomatico-orbital branch, which runs along the upper border of the zygomatic arch, between the two layers of the temporal fascia, to the lateral angle of the orbit. This branch, which may arise directly from the superficial temporal artery, supplies the orbicularis oculi, and anastomoses with the lacrimal and palpebral branches of the ophthalmic artery.
   - ***Anterior Auricular Branches:*** are distributed to the anterior portion of the auricula, the lobule, and part of the external acoustic meatus, anastomosing with the posterior auricular.
   - ***Frontal Branch:*** runs tortuously upward and forward to the forehead, supplying the muscles, integument, and pericranium in this region, and anastomosing with the supraorbital and frontal arteries.
   - ***Parietal Branch:*** larger than the frontal, curves upward and backward on the side of the head, lying superficial to the temporal fascia, and anastomosing with its fellow of the opposite side, and with the posterior auricular and occipital arteries.

MAXILLARY ARTERY

This is the larger terminal branch of the external carotid artery, it is given off posteromedially to the neck of the mandible and deep to the anteromedial surface of the parotid gland.

COURSE AND RELATIONS

Divided into 3 parts by the lateral pterygoid muscle.

First part (or mandibular part)

Runs horizontally forwards, first between the neck of the mandible and the sphenomandibular ligament, below the auriculotemporal nerve, and then along the lower border of the lateral pterygoid.

Its branches pass through foramina:

- Deep auricular artery passes through a foramen between cartilagenous and bony external acoustic meatus supplies external acoustic meatus
- Anterior tympanic branch passes through medial and petro-tympanic fissure supplies (a) middle ear (b) medial surface of tympanic membrane
- Middle meningeal artery passes through foramen spinosum along with the meningeal branch of the mandibular nerve to middle cranial fossa.
- Accessory meningeal artery passes through foramen ovale to middle cranial fossa dura mater.
- Inferior alveolar artery passes through mandibular foramen accompanying the nerve of the same name and supplies mandibular teeth and alveoli.

Second Part (or pterygoid part)

Runs upwards and forwards either superficially or deep to lower head of lateral pterygoid:

Gives mainly muscular branches

- to pterygoid muscles (lateral and medial)
- deep temporal branches to temporalis muscle
- artery to the masseter muscle
- buccal artery to the buccinator muscle

Third Part (called pterygopalatine part)

Passes between 2 heads of lateral pterygoid and through the pterygomaxillary fissure, enters pterygopalatine fossa, lies in front pterygopalatine ganglion.

The third part gives off 6 branches.

- Posterior superior alveolar artery. Descends on the posterior surface of the maxilla and gives branches that enter canals in the bone and supplies the molar and premolar teeth and the antrum of Highmore (maxillary air sinus).

- Infraorbital artery enters the orbit through the inferior orbital fissure, runs forwards on the floor of the orbit, first in the infraorbital groove, in infraorbital canal to emerge on the face through the infraorbital foramen. It branches orbital anterior superior alveolar branches that enter apertures in the maxilla to reach the incisor and canine teeth. In the face the infraorbital artery gives nasal, labial and palpebral branches.
- Greater palatine artery runs through the greater palatine foramen. It then runs forwards near the lateral margin of the palate to reach the incisive canal (near the midline) through which some terminal branches enter the nasal cavity. Branches of the artery supply the palate and the gums. While still within the greater palatine canal it gives off the lesser palatine arteries that emerge on the palate through the lesser palatineforamina, and run backwards into the soft palate and tonsil.
- Pharyngeal branch runs backwards through palatinovaginal canal. It supplies part of the nasopharynx, the auditory tube and the sphenoidal air sinuses.
- Artery of the pterygoid canal runs backwards in the canal of the same name and supplies the pharynx, the auditory tube and the middle ear.
- Sphenopalatine artery passes through the foramen of the same name to enter the cavity of the nose. Gives off posterolateral nasal branches; and posterior septal branches to the nasal septum.

In Sum it supplies:

- the upper and lower jaws (all maxillary and mandibular teeth)
- the dura mater
- the external and middle ears, and the auditory tube
- the muscles of the temporal and infratemporal fossa (all masticatory muscles)
- the nose and paranasal air sinuses
- the palate
- the roof of the pharynx.

14
Veins of Head and Neck

VEINS

- **Frontal vein:** begins on the forehead in a venous plexus which communicates with the frontal branches of the superficial temporal vein. The veins converge to form a single trunk, which runs downward near the middle line of the forehead parallel with the vein of the opposite side. At the root of the nose the veins diverge, and, each at the medial angle of the orbit. Joins the supraorbital vein, to form the angular vein.
- **Supraorbital vein:** begins on the forehead where it communicates with the frontal branch of the superficial temporal vein. It runs downward superficial to the frontalis muscle, and joins the frontal vein at the medial angle of the orbit to form the angular vein. Before its junction with the frontal vein, it sends a branch which communicates with the ophthalmic vein through the supraorbital notch into the orbit; as this

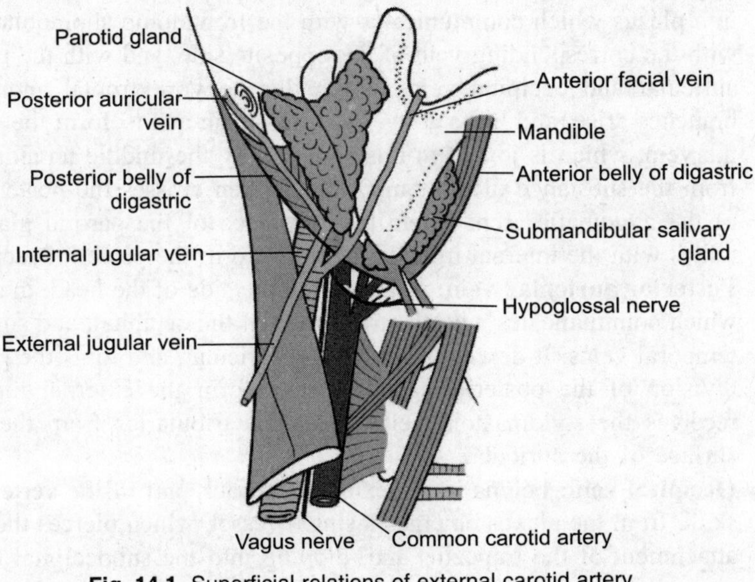

Fig. 14.1. Superficial relations of external carotid artery.

vessel passes through the notch, it receives the frontal diploic vein through a foramen at the bottom of the notch.

- **Angular vein:** formed by the junction of the frontal and supraorbital veins, runs obliquely downward, on the side of the root of the nose, to the level of the lower margin of the orbit, where it becomes the anterior facial vein. It receives the veins of the ala nasi, and communicates with the superior ophthalmic vein through the nasofrontal vein, thus establishing an important anastomosis between the anterior facial vein and the cavernous sinus.
- **Anterior facial vein:** commences at the side of the root of the nose, and is a direct continuation of the angular vein. It lies behind the external maxillary (facial) artey and follows a less tortuous course. It runs oblique downward and backward, beneath the Zygomatic and zugomatic head of the Quadratus labii superioris, descends along the anterior border and then on the superficial surface of the masseter, crosses over the body of the mandible, and passes obliquely backward, beneath the platysma and cervical fascia, superficial to the submandibular gland, the digastic and stylohyoid. It unites with the posterior facial vein to form the common facial vein, which crosses the external carotid artey and enters the internal jugular vein at a variable point below the hyoid bone. From near its termination a communicating branch often runs down the anterior border of the sternocleidomastoid to join the lower part of the anterior jugular vein. The facial vein has no valves, and its walls are not so flaccid as most superficial veins.
- **Superficial temporal vein:** begins on the side and vertex of the skull in a plezus which communicates with the frontal and supraobital veins, with the corresponding vein of the opposite side, and with the posterior auricular and occipital veins. From this network frontal and parietal branches arise, and unite above the zygomatic ach to form the trunk of the vein, which is joined in this situation by the middle temporal vein, from the substance of the temporalis. It then crosses the posterior root of the zygomatic arch, enters the substance of the parotid gland, and unites with the internal maxillary vein to form the posterior facial vein.
- **Posterior auricular vein:** Begins upon the side of the head, in a plexus which communicates with the tributaries of the occipital, and superficial temporal veins. It descends behind the auricular, and joins the posterior division of the posterior facial vein to form the external jugular. It receives the stylomastoid vein, and some tributaries from the cranial surface of the auricular.
- **Occipital vein:** begins in a plexus at the back part of the vertex of the skull, from the plexus emerges a single vessel, which pierces the cranial attachment of the trapezius and, dipping into the suboccipital triangle,

join the deep cervical and vertebral veins. Occasionally it follows the course of the occipital artey and ends in the internal jugular; in other instances, it joins the posterior auricular and through it opens into the external jugular. The parietal emissary vein connects it with the superior sagittal sinus; and as it passes across the mastoid portion of the temporal bone, it receives the mastoid emissary vein which connects it with the transverse sinus. The occipital diploic vein sometimes joins it.

- **Internal maxillary vein:** is a short trunk which accompanies the first part of the internal maxillary artery. It is formed by a confluence of the veins of the pterygoid plexus, and passes backward between the sphenomandibular ligament and the neck of the mandible, and unites with the temporal vein to form the posterior facial vein.
- **Posterior facial vein:** formed by the union of the superficial and internal maxillary vein, descends in the substance of the parotid gland, superficial to the external carotid artery but beneath the facial nerve, between the branches, an anterior, which passes forward and unites with the anterior facial vein to form the common facial vein and a posterior, which is joined by the posterior auricular vein and becomes the external vein.
- **Pterygoid venous plexus:** is of considerable size, and is situated between the temporalis and pterygoid, and partly between the two pterygoids. It receives tributaries corresponding with the branches of the internal maxillary artery. Thus it receives the sphenopalatine, the middle meningeal, the deep temporal, the pterygoid, massesteric, buccinator, alveolar, and some palatine veins, and a branch which communicates with the ophthalmic vein through the inferior orbital fissure. This plexus communicates freely with the anterior facial vein; it also communicates with the cavernous sinus, by branches through the foramen vesalii, foramen ovale, and foramen lacerum.

15

Craniometry: Anthropometry of the Skull

Physical anthropologists have used certain points and anatomical landmarks between which measurements are made. In recent years , many anthropometric methods and terms have been adopted in specialized dental fields such as orthodontia. It may , however , be noted that measurements made in the living differ in a number of respects from those made on the skeleton. Nevertheless, it seems desirable, not only to enumerate and define certain points and lines of measurement on the skull, but to discuss briefly those that are most useful to the dentist (Shapiro,1947). Bony landmarks that can easily be seen or palpated through the soft tissues on the surface are shown in figure.

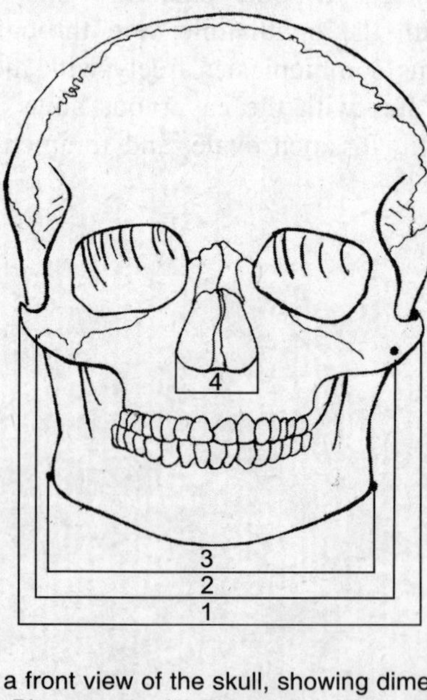

Fig. 15.1. Diagram of a front view of the skull, showing dimensions in width of facial features: (1) Bizygomatic, (2) Bicondylar, (3) bigonial, (4) Nasal.

- ***The alveolar point :*** the lowest point of the upper alveolar process (of maxilla) found at the gingival level between the upper central incisors.
- ***The auricular point or auriculare:*** is located at the centre of the opening of the external acoustic meatus.The roof of the opening, is named porion, is also often used as a point of reference.
- ***The glabella :*** is a smooth prominence located on the frontal lobe just above the root of the nose, on a level with the superior orbital margin.
- ***The condylar point :*** is the most prominent point on the outer surface of the head of the mandibular condyle and is palpable just anterior to the tragus of the ear. It is commonly used by prosthodontists.
- ***The glenoid point :*** is located at the centre of the glenoid fossa of the temporal bone. The outer border of this fossa can be palpated just above the mandibular condyle and is readily determined when the mouth is opened, by pressing a finger in the hollow caused by the withdrawal of the condylar head.
- ***Gonion :*** is the point of the angle formed by the ramus and body of the mandible. The outer surface of this angle can be easily palpated. But in some cases, it is more easily located when the mandible is protruded.
- ***The inferior alveolar point :*** is located at the gingival level of the lower anterior teeth between the central incisors (and is taken in the midline of the lower jaw if no incisors are present).
- ***The infraorbital point or orbitale:*** is the lowest point of the inferior orbital margin. It is located by exerting digital pressure along the inferior margin of orbit. This is the anterior point through which the Frankfurt plane passes (the latter being defined when the left and right Portia roof of external acoustic meatus and the left orbit is in the same horizontal plane.

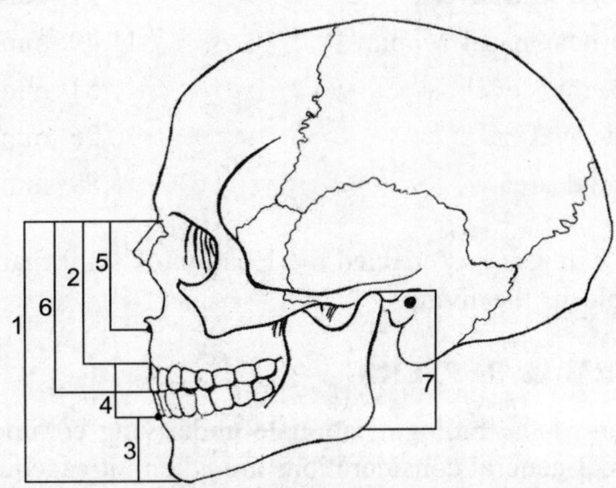

Fig. 15.2. Diagram of the skull, showing dimensions in height of facial features: (1) Total face, (2) Upper face, (3) Lower face, (4) Dental, (5) Nasal, (6) Nasio-incision, (7) Ramus.

- **The malar (zygomatic) point:** is the most prominent location on the zygomatic bone.
- **The mastoid point:** is located at the tip of mastoid process of temporal bone. It lies just below and posterior to the external acoustic meatus, palpable behind posterior border of the ramus of mandible.
- **The maximum occipital point:** is the point on the squamous part of occipital which is found to be the most distant from glabella.
- **The mental point, menton or gnathion:** is the most anterior point of the symphysis of mandible. But the vertical measurement of the face, the lowest or inferior mental point is chosen.
- **Nasion:** is the midpoint of nasal and frontal suture and found by pressure of a fingertip on the nasofrontal suture.
- **The subnasal point:** is located at the root of the nasal spine in the midline and can be palpated by digital pressure at the base of the nose.
- **The zygomatic-frontal point:** can be felt on the lateral margin of the orbit at the junction of the zygomatic and frontal bones.

Locating anthropometric points of the skull :

- **By palpation:** the ease of palpation is limited by the thickness of the overlying structures. The mental point, for instance, can be covered by a heavy layer of musculature and fatty tisuue. In an instructive paper, Krogman refers to certain local tissue thickness in the head region, and lists average tissue depths at various parts of the face in well nourished individuals as follows:

Forehead at the hairline	:	6.06 mm
Forehead at the mid-level	:	5.10 mm
Roof of the nose	:	5.55 mm
Nasal bridge mid-level	:	3.37 mm
Upper lip near nasal septum	:	11.49 mm
Upper lip, mid-level	:	9.51 mm
Chin, mid-level	:	10.26 mm
Supra orbital area	:	5.89 mm

- By X-ray : its use has enabled the location of skull markings hidden or inaccessible in the living.

FACIAL FORM & PATTERN

For description of the biologic rationale underlying common variations in facial features, 3 general considerations are taken into account:

- Different facial types as they relate to variations in the development of of overall form and shape of the whole head.

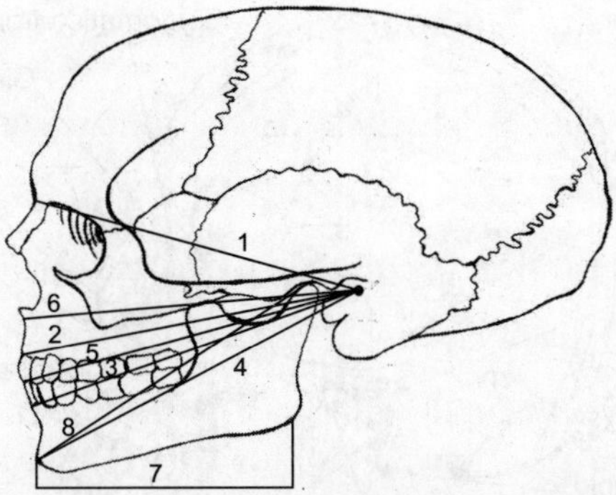

Fig. 15.3. Diagram showing dimensions in depth of facial features: (1) Auriculo-nasion, (2) Auriculo-prosthion, (3) Auriculo-infradental, (4) Auriculo-menton, (5) Auriculo-incision, (6) Auriculo-infranasal, (7) Gonio-menton, (8) Condylo-menton.

- Male and female developmental facial differences.
- Child and adult facial differences.

HEAD FORM

- Dolicocephalic Head Form: sets up a developing face that becomes corresponding narrow, long and protrusive. Facial type is termed leptoproscopic. Upper part of dolicocephalic nose is quite protrusive, the nose sometimes "bends" to produce an AQUILINE ("Roman or Dick Tracy") type of convex nasal contour, and the end of the more pointed nose frequently tips down (the effect increases as age advances).

  The dolicocephalic head form has a cranial index of 0.75 or less. Face is more angular and less flat. Mid face and the "open" (obtuse) form of its basicranial flexure relate to a downward-backward rotational alignment of the mandible. This results in a tendency for a retrusively placed mandible and retrusive lower lip with a retrognathic (convex) facial profile.

- **BRACHYCEPHALIC HEAD FORM:** establishes a face that is more broad, but somewhat less protrusive and this is called europroscopic facial type. Brachycephalic nose is pug like vertically and protrusively shorter, and it has a more rounded tip. The cranial index is 0.80 or greater. The eyeballs are characteristically more exopthalmic (proptopic). Face relates to a more "closed basicranial flexure". As a result the lower jaw tends to be variably more protrusive, with a greater tendency for a straighter or even concave facial profile and a more prominent appearance of the chin.
- **THE DINARIC HEAD FORM:** is a "brachycephalized dolicocephalic" having a long face and a large nose. It is primarily the

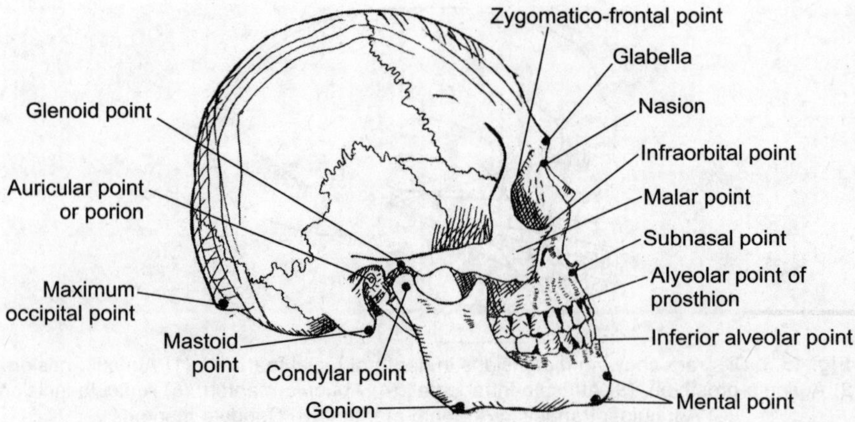

Fig. 15.4. Diagram of the skull, showing anthropometric landmarks.

posterior part of the dinaric head that has been brachycephalized. The occipital or lambdoidal regions become widened and markedly flattened, with bilateral peaking (bossing) of the parietal region. The ears of the dinaric form appear much closer to the back of the head because of the occipital flattening.The form of the face is distinctively leptoproscopic, quite unlike the typical europroscopic brachycephalic pattern. The nose tends to be very large and often aquiline and the nasal bridge is high. The mandible tends to be less retrusive, the face less retrognathic and the profile tending more toward orthognathic.

16
Meninges

MENINGES

(In a Membrane surrounding the CNS components i.e. brain and spinal cord)

The tough dura mater contains venous sinus (between the outer, endosteal layer and the inner, meningeal layer)

THE MENINGEAL LAYER

It is called falx cerebi because it is sickle-shaped, and is a strong, arched process which descends vertically in the longitudinal fissure between the cerebral hemispheres. It is narrow in front, where it is attached to the crista falli of the ethmoid; and broad behind, where it is connected with the upper surface of the tentorium cerebelli. Its upper margin is convex, and attached to the inner surface of the skull in the middle line, as far back as the internal occipital protuberance; it contains the superior sagittal sinus. Its lower margin is free and concave, and contains the inferior sagittal sinus.

Tentorium cerebelli is an arched lamina, elevated in the middle, and inclining downward towards the circumference. It covers the superior surface of the cerebellum, and supports the occipital lobes of the brain. Its anterior border is free and concave, and bounds a large over opening, the incisura tentorii, for the transmission of the cerebral peduncles. It is attached, behind, by its convex border, and there encloses ridges upon the inner surface of the occipital bone, and there encloses the transverse sinuses in front, to the superior angle of the petrous part of the temporal bone on either side, enclosing the superior petrosal sinuses. At the apex of the petrous part of the temporal bone the free and attached borders meet, and, crossing one another, are continued forward to be fixed to the anterior and posterior clinoid processes respectively. To the middle line of its upper surface the posterior border of the falx respectively. To the middle line of its upper surface the posterior border of the falx cerebri is attached, the straight sinus being placed at their line of junction.

Falx cerebelli is a small triangular process of dura mater, received into the posterior cerebellar notch. Its base is attached, above, to the under and back part of the tentorium; its posterior margin, to the lower division of the vertical crest on the inner surface of the occipital bone. As it descends, it sometimes divides into two smaller folds, which may be separated by an interval of 5mm **(as stated by Hasan and Das 1969 in the gray's anatomy)**

Diphragma sellae is a small circular horizontal fold, which roods in the sells turcica and almost completely covers the hypophysis; a small central opening transmits the infundibulm.

17

Dural Venous Sinuses

Cavernous sinuses are so named because they present a reticulated structure, due to their being traversed by numerous interlacing filaments. They are of irregular form, larger behind than in front, and are placed one on either side of the body of the sphenoid bone, extending from the superior orbital fissure to the apex of the petrous portion of the temporal bone. Each opens behind into the petrosal sinuses. On the medial wall of each sinus is the internal carotid artey, accompanied by filaments of the carotid plexus; near the artery is the abducent nerve; on the lateral wall are the oculomotor and trochelar nerves, and the ophthalmic and maxillary divisions of the trigeminal nerve. These structures are separated from the blood flowing along the sinus by the lining membrane of the sinus. The cavernous sinus receives the superior ophthalmic vein through the superior orbital fissure, some of the cerebral veins, and also the small sphenorietal sinus, which courses along the under surface of the small wing of the sphenoid. It communicates with the transverse sinus by means of the superior petrosal sinus; with the internal jugular vein through the inferior petrosal sinus and a plexus of veins on the internal carotid artery; with pterygoid venous plexus through the foramen vesalii, foramen ovale, and foramen lacerum, and with the angular vein through the ophthalmic vein. The two sinuses also communicate with each other by means of the anterior and posterior intercavernous sinuses.

RELATIONS

Intercavernous sinuses

Intercavernous sinuses are two in number, an anterior and a posterior, and connect the two cavernous sinuses across the middle line. The anterior passes in front of the hypophysis cerebri, the posterior behind it, and they form with the cavernous sinuses a vernous circle (circular sinus) around the hypophysis. The anterior one is usually the large of the two, and one or other is occasionally absent.

Superior Sagittal Sinus

Superior sagittal sinus occupies the attached or convex margin of the falx cerebri. Commencing at the foramen caecum, through which it receives a vein from the nasal cavity, it runs from before backward, grooving the inner surface of the frontal, the adjacent margins of the two parietals, and the superior division of the cruciate eminence of the occipital; near the internal occipital protuberance it deviates to one or other side (usually the right), and is continued as the corresponding transverse sinus. It is triangular in section, narrow in front, and gradually increases in size as it passes backward. Its inner surface presents the openings of the superior cerebral veins, which run, for the most part, obliquely forward, and open chiefly at the back part of the sinus, their orifices being concealed by fibrous; numerous fibrous bands extend **transversely across.**

The inferior angle of the sinus; and, lastly, small opening communicate with irregularly shaped venous spaces (venous lacunae) in the dura mater near the sinus. There are usually three lacunae on either side of the sinus; a small frontal, a large parietal, and an occipital, intermediate in size between the other two. Most of the cerebral veins from the outer surface of the hemisphere open into these lacunae, and numerous arachnoid granulations project into them from below. The superior sagittal sinus receives the superior cerebral veins, veins from the dipole and dura mater, and near the posterior extremity of the sagittal suture, veins from the pericranium, which pass through the parietal foramina. The numerous communications exist between this sinus and the veins of the nose, scalp and diploe.

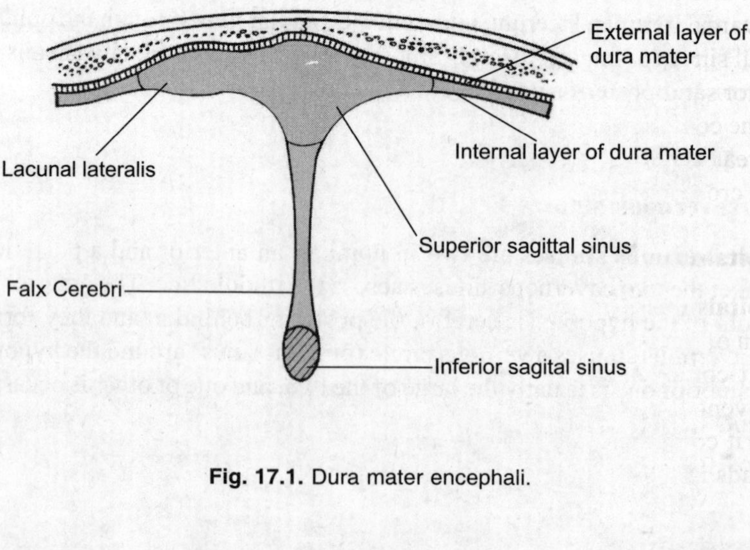

Fig. 17.1. Dura mater encephali.

Inferior sagittal sinus

Inferior sagittal sinus is contained in the posterior half or two-thirds of the free margin of the falx cerebri. It is a cylindrical form, increases in size as it passes backward, and ends in the straight sinus. It receives several veins from the falx cerebri, and occasionally a few from the medial surface of the hemispheres.

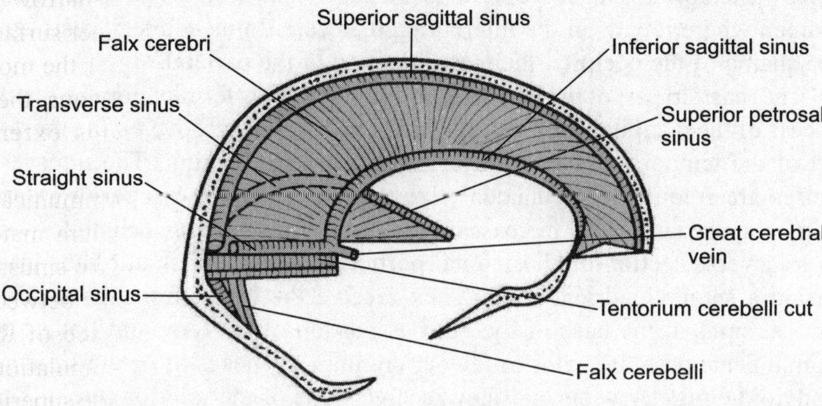

Fig. 17.2. Dural venous sinuses. Tentorium removed on one side to expose falx cerebelli.

Straight sinus

Straight sinus is situated at the line of junction of the falx cerebri with the tentorium cerevelli. It is triangular in section, increases in size as it proceeds backward, and runs downward and backward from the end of the inferior sagittal sinus to the transverse sinus of the opposite side to that into which the superior sagittal sinus is prolonged. Its terminal part communicates by a cross with the confluence of the sinuses. Besides the inferior sagittal sinus, it receives the great cerebral vein and the superior cerebellar veins. A few transverse bands cross its interior.

Occipitalsinus

Occipitalsinus is the smallest of the cranial sinuses. It is situated in the attached margin of the falx cerebelli, and is generally single, but occasionally there are two. It commences around the margin of the foramen magnum by several small venous channels, one of which joins the terminal part of the transverse sinus; it communicates with the posterior internal vertebral venous plexuses and ends in the confluence of the sinuses.

Transverse sinuses

Transverse sinuses are of large size and begin at the internal occipital protuberance; one, generally the right, being the direct continuation of the superior sagittal sinus, the other of the straight sinus. Each transverse sinus passes lateralward and forward, describing a slight curve with its convexity upward, to the base of the petrous portion of the temporal bone, and lies in this part of its course in the attached margin of the tentorium cerebelli; it then leaves the tentorium and curves downward and medialward to reach the jugular foramen where it ends in the internal jugular vein. In its course it rests upon the squama of the occipital the mastoid angle of the parietal.

The mastoid part of the temporal and just before its termination the jugular process of the occipital the portion which occupies the groove on the mastoid part of the temporal is sometimes termed the sigmoid sinus.The transverse sinuses are frequently of unequal size that formed by the superior sagittal sinus being the larger they increase in size as they proceed from behind forward. On transverse section the horizontal portion exhibits a prismatic the curved portion a semicylendrical form. They receive the blood from the superior petrosal sinus at the base of the petrous portion of the temporal bone; they communicate with the veins of the pericranium by means of the mastoid and condyloid emissary veins and they receive some of the inferior cerebral and inferior cerebellar veins and some veins from the diploe. The petrosquamous sinus when present runs backward along the junction of the squama and petrous portion of the temporal and opens into the transverse sinus.

Superior petrosal sinus

Superior petrosal sinus small and narrow connects the cavernous with the transverse sinus. It runs lateralward backward from the posterior end of the cavernous sinus over the trigeminal nerve and lies in the attached margin of the tentorium cerebelli and in the superior petrosal sulcus of the temporal bone it joins the transverse sinus where the latter curves downward on the inner surface of the mastoid part of the temporal. It receives some cerebellar and inferior cerebral veins and veins from the tympanic cavity.

Inferior petrosal sinus

Inferior petrosal sinus is situated in the inferior petrosal sulcus formed by the junction of the petrous part of the temporal with the basilar part of the occipital begins in the postero-inferior part of the cavernous sinus and passing through the anterior part of the jugular foramen it ends in the superior bullb of the internal jugular vein. The inferior petrosal sinus receives the internal auditory veins and the veins from the medulla oblongata pons and undersurface of the cerebellum.

Emissary Veins

The emissary veins pass through apertures in the cranial wall and establish communication between the sinus inside the skull and the vein external to it. Some are always present others only occasionally so.

The principal emissary veins are the following:

1. A mastoid emissary vein usually present runs through the mastoid foramen and unites the transverse sinus with the posterior auricular or with the occipital vein.
2. A parietal emissary vein passes through the parietal foramen and connects the superior sagittal sinus with the veins of the scalp.
3. A network of minute veins traverses the hypoglossal canal and joins the transverse sinus with the vertebral vein and deep veins of the neck.
4. An inconstant condyloid emissary vein passes through the conduloid canal and connects the transverse sinus with the deep veins of the neck.
5. A network of veins unites the cavernous since with the pterygoid plexus through the foramen ovale.
6. Two or three small veins run through the foramen lacerum and connect the cavernous sinus with the pterygoid plexus.
7. The emissary vein of the foramen of vesalius connects the same parts.
8. An internal carotid plexus of veins traverses the carotid canal and unites the cavernous sinus with the internal jugular vein.
9. A vein is transmitted through the foramen cecum and connects the superior sagittal sinus with the veins of the nasal cavity.

18
Cavernous Sinus

CAVERNOUS SINUS

Paired venous sinuses enclosed between the inner and outer layer of dura mater.

- Location : situated on either side of the hypophyseal fossa of the body of the sphenoid bone, in the middle cranial fossa.
- Dimension : 2×1cm
- Structure : criss-cross fibrous septa divide it into a number of endothelial lined "honey-comb" like space (little caverns). Hence its name "cavernous sinus.
- Extent : Anteriorly – upto medial end of superior orbital fissure.
  Posteriorly – upto apex of petrous temporal bone
  Medially – side of body of sphenoid
  Laterally – upto a sagittal plane just medial to the foramen ovale.

RELATIONS

(I) Outside the wall of sinus

- Medially
  - At a lower palne sphenoidal air sinus
  - At a higher plane hypophysis cerebri
- Laterally
  - Uncus of temporal lobe of cerebral hemisphere
  - Trigeminal ganglion and mandibular nerve
- Superiorly
  - Terminal part of internal carotid artery
  - Optic tract
- Inferiorly
  - Junction of greater wing of sphenoid with body of sphenoid
  - Foramen lacerum
- Anteriorly
  - Medial end of superior orbital fissure

- Posteriorly
  – Junction of pons with midbrain

(II) Relations within the wall of the cavernous sinus

- In the lateral wall from above downwards oculomotor nerve, trochlear nerve, ophthalmic division of Vth CN, maxillary division of Vth CN
- Inside cavernous sinus runs internal carotid artery surrounded by a plexus of sympathetic nerves (separated from the blood in the sinus by endothelial lining). Inferolateral to internal carotid artery runs the abducent nerve.

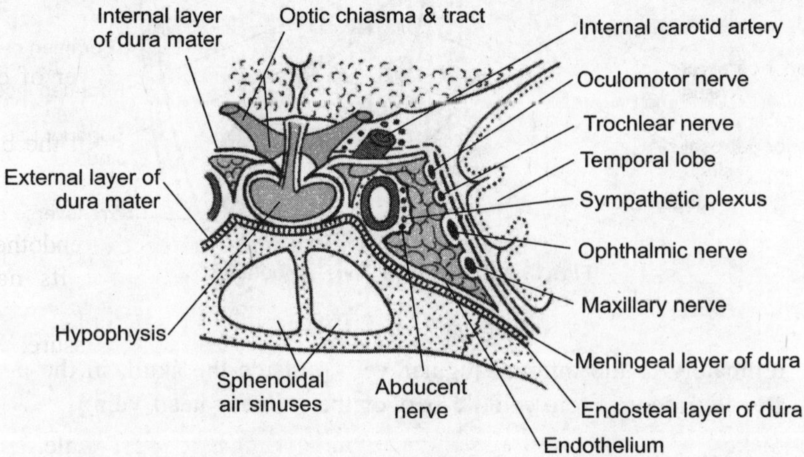

Fig. 18.1. Cavernous sinus—relations and contents.

TRIBUTARIES OF CAVERNOUS SINUS

- **Anteriorly:** superior and inferior ophthalmic veins
- **Medially:** Anteriorly and posterior intercavernous sinuses connect the 2 cavernous sinuses. Hypophyseal vein drains into the cavernous sinus. They form a "circular sinus" with 2 cavernous sinuses.
- **Laterally:** Middle meningeal vein communicates
- **Superiorly:** superficial middle cerebral vein and some inferior cerebral veins join it.
- **Inferiorly:** emissary veins passing through foramen lacerum (from pterygoid venous plexus).
- **Posterioly:** (1) Superior petrosal sinus drains into the junction of transverse and sigmoid sinuses (2) Inferior petrosal sinus (passes through jugular foramen to drain into the superior bulb of internal jugular vein extracranially). Thus the blood from cavernous sinus drains posteriorly,

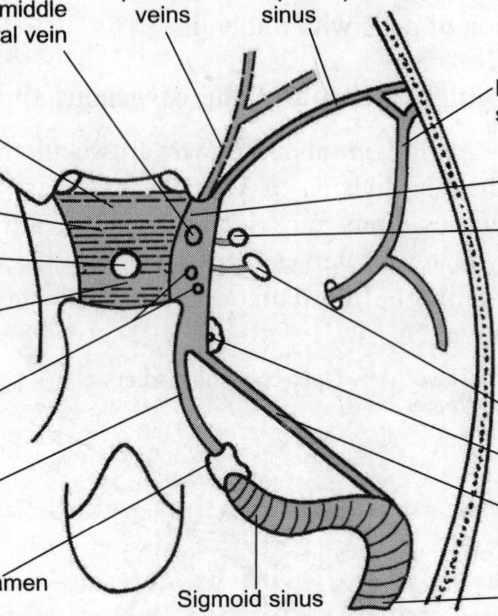

Fig. 18.2. Cavernous sinus—tributaries.

ultimately to the internal jugular vein (outside the skull, in the neck)

- **Development:** From middle part of the primary head vein.

APPLIED ANATOMY

- The cavernous sinus is connected to facial vein via ophthalmic veins directly and via emissary veins – pterygoid plexus
  - deep facial vein – facial vein indirectly. Thus a pustule in the "danger triangle of the face" if squeezed, infective emboli may travel to the cavernous sinus causing cavernous sinus thrombosis.
- Root abscess of canine tooth if not timely treated with appropriate antibiotics may cause infective thrombosis of facial vein and he emboli may travel via the above-mentioned routes to cavernous sinus, leading to dangerous thrombosis of this sinus which may be fatal.

Physical signs of cavernous sinus thrombosis include early involvement of abducent running through it postero-anteriorly (convergent squint of eye of that side due to unopposed action of medial rectus when lateral rectus is consequently paralysed). Also, paralysis of all other muscles of eyeball (due to involvement of IIIrd and IVth nerves running in the lateral wall) follows.

19

Thyroid Gland

THYROID GLAND

It lies in front in the anterior triangle of the neck covering the thyroid cartilage, cricoid cartilage and the 2,3,4 tracheal ring, normally weighs about 25 grams.

The gland has two lobes, shaped roughly like a pear. The right lobe is often larger than the left lobe and both are joined by a narrow isthmus on the anterior surface of the trachea. Sometimes a small pyramidal lobe arises from the isthmus somewhere along its upper border near the midline.

RELATIONS

Anterolateral overlaid by sternocleidomastoid muscle deep to which it is covered by the sternohyoid and the sternothyroid and laterally by the omohyoid muscle.

Posterior overlaps the carotid sheath behind which passes

Medial 2 cartilages   Thyroid cartilage
                       Cricoid cartilage

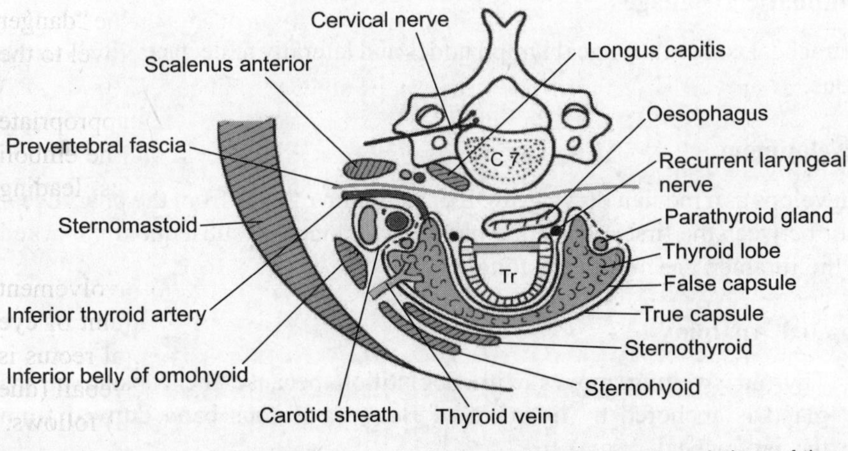

Fig. 19.1. T.S. through neck at the level of C7 vertebra to show the relations of thyroid gland.

2 tubes	Trachea
	Oesophagus
2 muscle	Cricothyroid
	Inferior constrictor of pharynx
2 membrane	Cricothyroid
	Cricotracheal
2 nerve	External laryngeal nerve
	Recurrent laryngeal nerve

ARTERIAL SUPPLY

- Superior thyroid artery branch of the external carotid artery
- Inferior thyroid artery branch of thyrocervical trunk given by the subclavian artery
- Arteria thyroidea ima unpaired and single branch of brachiocephalic or arch of aorta
- Accessory thyroid artery from trachea and oesophagus.

VENOUS DRAINAGE

- Superior thyroid vein which opens into the internal jugular vein.
- Middle hyoid vein which opens into the internal jugular vein.
- Inferior thyroid vein goes down to thorax into the left brachiocephalic vein
- Sometimes there is a 4th thyroid vein running directly into the internal jugular vein.

NERVE SUPPLY

Lymphatic Drainage

Pretracheal and prelaryngeal lymph nodes and laterally to deep cervical lymph nodes.

Development

It develops as a median down growth of a column of cells from the pharyngeal floor between the first and second pharyngeal pouches (subsequently marked by the foramen caecum of the tongue).

Applied Anatomy

- Thyroid swelling moves with deglutition because the capsule of the gland is anchored by ligament of Berry (a fibrous band derived from the pretracheal fascia)

- Arteries are ligatured or tied between 2 capsules when the gland is removed (thyroidectomy) the false capsule is left in the body.
- Superior thyroid artery should be ligatured as close to the upper pole as possible to avoid the inclusion of the external laryngeal nerve.
- Inferior thyroid artery should be toed as far away as possible from the gland to avoid injury to recurrent laryngeal nerve.
- Ectopic thyroid may lie elsewhere other than its normal location.
- Thyroglossal cyst results from the persistence of the thyroglossal duct
- Total agenesis of one lobe may occur but it is rare.

PARATHYROID GLAND

The number of the parathyroids vary from 2 to 6 but in 80 percent of cases, there are 4 (2 on each side). The total weight of 4 normal glands is about 140 mg

Embryology

The upper parathyroids arise from the 4th branchial pouch and come to lie in close association with the upper part of the lateral lobes of the thyroid. This position is constant. The lower parathyroids arise from the 3rd branchial pouch in association with the thymus, and descends with the thymus. Because of the embryological migration they may be found anywhere from the upper pole of the thyroid to the anterior mediastinum.

Anatomy

The glands are the size of a split pea. They are pink or brown in colour, but are frequently covered by fat, making them difficult to recognize. The superior gland lies on the posterior surface of the middle third of the thyroid, usually above the inferior thyroid artery, but well posterior to this plane. If enlarged they may descend into the posterior mediastinum. The inferior glands are mostly found on the posterior surface of the lower pole of the thyroid or within 1 cm below the lower pole. They may be higher or lower, occasionally as far down as in the thymus in the anterior mediastinum. They lie in a more anterior plane than the upper glands.

OSTEOLOGY

20
Nerve Supply of Muscles of Head & Neck at a Glance

All mucles of the tongue (end in – glossus), are supplied by the Hypoglossal nerve (XII C.N.) except:

Palatoglossus, which is supplied by cranial accessory via vagus through pharyngeal plexus which supplies all the muscles of pharynx, larynx and soft palate except:

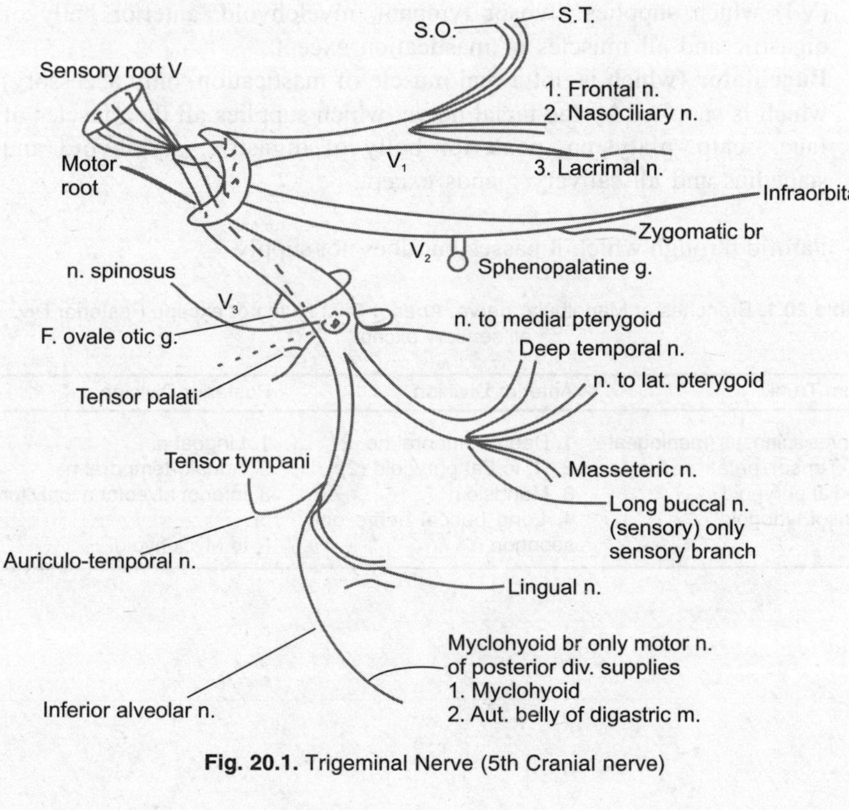

Fig. 20.1. Trigeminal Nerve (5th Cranial nerve)

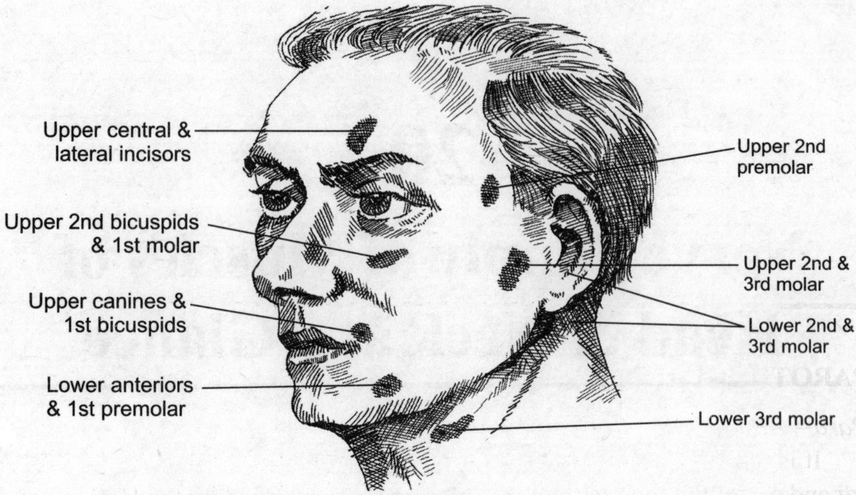

Fig. 20.2.

Tensor Palati, which is supplied by mandibular division of trigeminal (V3) which supplies: Tensor tympani, myelohyoid, anterior belly of digastric and all muscles of mastication except:
Buccinator (which is not a real muscle of mastication, only accessory) which is supplied by the facial nerve, which supplies all the muscles of face, scalp, platysma, posterior belly of digastric, stylohyoid and stapedius and all salivary glands except.

Parotid through which it passes but does not supply.

Table 20.1. Branches of Mandibular nerve. Anerior Div.: all motor except, Posterior Div.: all sensory except.

From Trunk	Anterior Division	Posterior Division
Nerves spinosus (meningeal br. Tensor palati nerve to medial phrygoid Tensor tyhogoid	1. Deep Temporal ne. 2 2. N. to Lat phrygoid (2) 3. Mandsic n 4. Long buccal nerve only seongon n.	1. Lingual n. 2. Aurialo-temporal n 3. Inferior alveolor n. only for br. N to Myclohyoid.

21

Parotid Gland

PAROTID GLAND

Para= Beside, Otis=Ear (gland located beside ear)

It is the largest salivary gland, weighing around 25g.It lies by the side of ear and in front of the ear, in the posterior part of the face, between the mastoid process and the ramus of mandible.

DIAGRAM

Styloid Apparatus

Ligament

- Stylomandibular ligament
- Stylohyoid ligament

Muscle

- Styloglossus muscle
- Stylopharyngeus muscle
- Stylohyoid muscle

DIAGRAM

Surfaces	Borders
1. Superior surface (Concave)	1. Posterior Border
2. Lateral surface (Superficial)	2. Anterior Border
	3. Medial Border

Veins of neck = Jugular
Arteries of Neck = Carotid

PAROTID GLAND – Shape
- Irregular
- Inverted Pyramidal

Borders	Surfaces
1. Anterior 2. Posterior 3. Medial **End** 1. Upper 2. Lower	1. Superficial or lateral surface 2. Anteromedial 3. Posteromedial 4. Superior

RELATIONS

Lower end paroid descends into neck carotid triangle and is crossed by platysma

Platysma- Subcutaneous muscle of neck, moves the skin of neck.

Neck Skin ————————————

Most Superficial→ ————————————

Platysma ————————————

Deep vessels and nerves

RELATIONS

ANTEROMEDIAL	POSTEROMEDIAL
1. Masseter 2. Mandible 3. Medial Pterygoid 4. Temporomandibular Joint 5. Branches of VIIth C N **SUPERIOR SURFACE** 1. External Acoustic Meatus **SUPERFICIAL OR LATERAL SURFACE** 1. Skin 2. Superficial Fascia 3. Auricular temporal nerve 4. Great Auricular 5. Platysma (lower end) 6. Superficial parotid lymph nodes 7. Deep Fascia	1. Sternocleidomastoid 2. Posterior belly of digastric 3. Mastoid process of temporal bone 4. Styloid Process 5. Stylohyoid 6. Styloglossus 7. Stylopharyngeus 8. Stylomandibular 9. Stylohyoid 10. Internal Carotid Artery 11. Internal Jugular Vein 12. Glossopharyngeal 13. Vagus 14. Accessory 15. Hypoglossal

Inside Parotid Gland (Relation) within the parotid gland: from superficial to deep:

1. Facial Nerve (nerve is nearer to the skin)
2. Retromandible
3. External Carotid Artery
4. Deep Parotid lymph nodes (scattered)

PAROTID GLAND

1. Accessory Parotid in some cases (about 30%)
2. Glenoid Process (temporomandibular joint)
3. Pterygoid Process (between medial pterygoid and the ramus of mandible)

DIAGRAM

Opening of Parotid duct:

It is at a raised papilla (nipple-like projection) at the level of crown of 2nd upper molar tooth in the vestibule of the mouth.

DIAGRAM

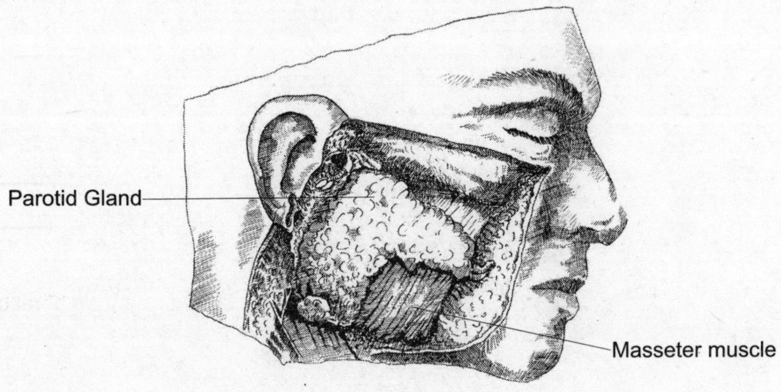

Fig. 21.1. Showing a dissection of the lateral aspect of the parotid gland.

Oral Cavity — Oral cavity proper / Vestibule of mouth

Buccina—Trumpet (wind based musical instrument)
Buccinator—used for blowing trumpet or other muscical instrument

1. ***Nerve Supply:*** Parasympathetic through 9th nerve and sympathetic fibres around external carotid artery.
2. ***Arterial Supply:*** branches of superficial temporal and maxillary artery (terminal branches of external carotid artery)
3. ***Venous Drainage:*** Retromandibular vein
4. ***Lymphatic Drainage:*** Parotid lymph nodes

APPLIED ANATOMY

1. Mumps is a viral disease causing inflamation (swelling) of the parotid gland.
2. Viral parotiditis is a painful swelling of the parotid gland.
3. In tumor of the parotid gland the superficial lobe lying superficial to the nerve can be removed (called superficial parotidectomy). The procedure of the removal of the entire parotid gland is called parotidectomy.

22

Submandibular Gland

SUBMANDIBULAR GLAND

The second largest salivary gland (after parotid) lies in the digastric/ submandibular triangle, partly under the cover of the posterior half of the body of mandible. Its contact with the bone causes smooth elongated concavity below the mylohyoid ridge opposite the premolars and molars. Almost the size of a walnut, it narrows posteriorly and curves around the posterior border of myelohyoid. The continuity into a small deep part which lies in the floor of mouth, between mandible and side of tongue (between myelohyoid and hyoglossus muscles). Thus it has a (i) large superficial part lodged in the neck. (ii) a small deep part, above the oral diaphragm (myelohyoid) in the oral cavity. The main duct of the gland (Wharton's Duct) emerges from the deep surface of the cervical superficial part of the gland and curves around the posterior border of myelohyoid (along with the deep part)

FASCIAL CAPSULE

The investing layer of the deep cervical fascia splits at its lower border to enclose the gland.

SURFACES OF THE GLAND

1. Infero-lateral
2. Lateral
3. Medial

RELATIONS

1. Inferolateral
   - Skin
   - Superficial fascia
   - Platysma
   - Mandibular branch of facial nerve
   - Facial vein

- Deep fascia (superficial part of capsule)
- Lymph nodes

2. Lateral surface
   - Submandibular fossa of mandible
   - Medial pterygoid muscle
   - Facial artery (loop)
3. Medial (deep) surface
   - Posteriorly : overlaps middle constrictor of pharynx, lingual artery and glossopharyngeal nerve
   - In the middle : comes hyoglossus muscle, styloglossus, lingual nerve, submandibular ganglion, hypoglossal nerve and vein accompanying it.
   - Anteriorly : myelohyoid, submental vessels, myelohyoid nerve and vessels.

Thus the deep surface covers 3 muscles (middle constrictor, hyoglossus and myelohyoid plus structures related to them.)

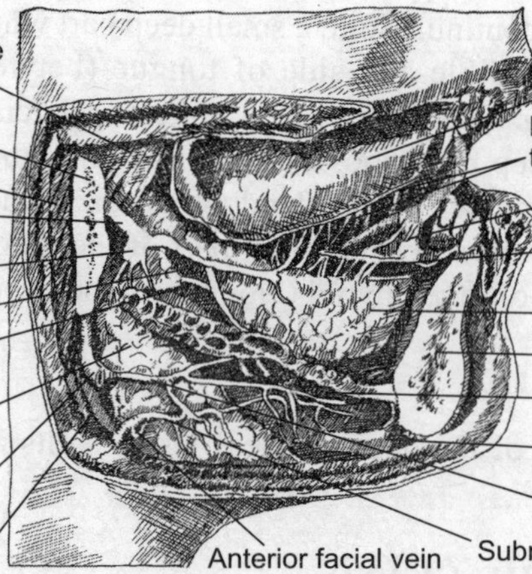

Fig. 22.1. Diagram showing the submandibular gland.

Deep part of Submandibular Gland

Tongue-shaped, insinuates between myelohyoid and hyoglossus and reaches upto sublingual gland. In the interval between the two, lingual nerve spirals around submandibular duct.

Nerve Supply

Secretomotor (parasympathetic) fibres from submandibular ganglion (the preganglionic branch) arises from the chorda tympani branch of facial nerve joining the lingual nerve from which hangs the submandibular ganglion).

Blood Supply

Facial artery and common facial vein.

Lymphatic Drainage

Lymphatic Drainage into submandibular lymph nodes and then into longitudinal drain (along internal jugular) of deep cervical lymph nodes.

DEVELOPMENT

A groove in the floor of mouth becomes converted into a tunnel whose posterior blind end proliferates to form the secretory acini. The original evagination gives rise to submandibular duct.

APPLIED ANATOMY

Submandibular lymphnodes are not only on lateral surface but are within the substance of the gland too. One outlying member lies in the loop of facial artery related to its lateral surface (called gland of Stohr) In cancers of the oral cavity or lips/cheek, These glands must be removed completely. For this purpose, the submandibualar gland itself has to be excised.

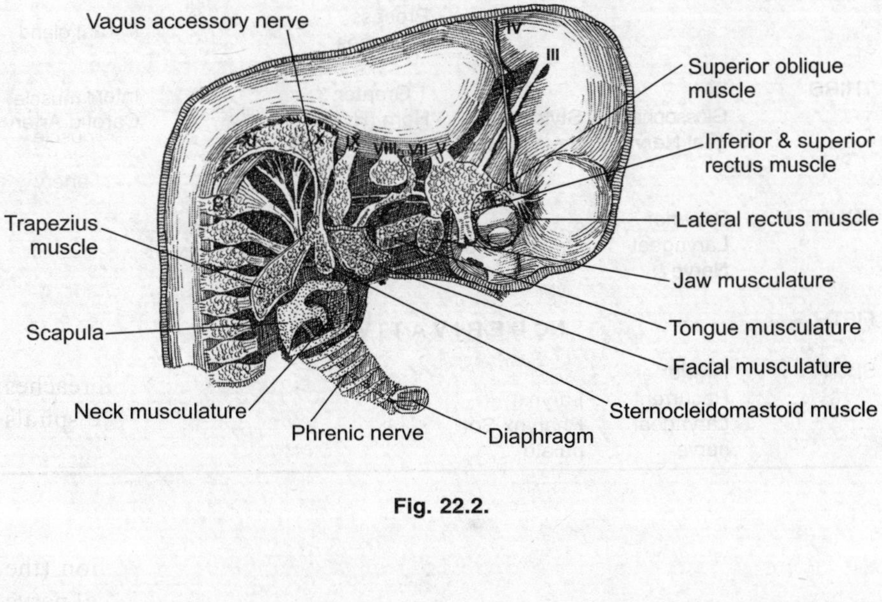

Fig. 22.2.

Structure Derived from Bronchial arches and their innervations

Arch	Nerve	Muscles	Skeletal Structure	Ligaments	Artery
FIRST (Mandibular)	Mandibular (V_3)	1. Muscles of mastication Temporalis, masseter, lateral & medial pterygoid 2. Myelohyoid & anterior belly of digastric 3. Tensor tympani & Tensor palati	1. Meckel's Cartilage (Membrane around this Cartilage gives rise to mandible 2. Zygomatic bone 3. Squamous part of temporal bone 4. Zygomatic arch 5. Malleus 6. Incus	1. Spheno-mandibular ligament 2.Anterior ligament of malleus	Disappears its remnant is maxillary artery
SECOND (Hyoid)	Seventh C.N.(Facial nerve)	1. Muscles of face, scalp & platysma 2. Stapedius 3. Stylohyoid 4. Posterior belly of digastric	Reichert's bar (Cartilage) 1. Superior Half of Hyloid 2. Smaller Cornua of (Horn) 3. Styloid Process 4. Stapes	Stylohyoid ligament	Disappears (Stapedial Artery)
THIRD	IX Glossopharyngeal Nerve	Stylopharyngeus Muscle	1.Greater Horn (Hyoid) 2. Inferior Half Body of Hyoid		Internal Carotid Artery
FOURTH	Superior Laryngeal Nerve	Cricothyroid	Thyroid Cartilage		
FIFTH		**NO DERIVATIVES**			
SIXTH	Inferior or Recurrent Laryngeal nerve	Larynx, Pharynx Soft palate			

23

Articulated Skull

Articulated Skull

Neurocranium (brain box) bones (8), enclosing cranial cavity, containing brain and meninges (coverings):

Paired	Unpaired
Paretal-2	Frontal-1
Temporal-2	Occipital-1
	Sphenoid-1
	Ethmoid-1

1. Vault (top) of cranium called calvaria composed of membrane bones (intra-membranous ossification)
2. Base of cranium chondrocranium = (ossified in cartilage)

Cranial cavity, rigid box contain brain, blood and cerebrospinal fluid (CSF)

Valveless emissary veins passing through cranial foramina. Communicate intracranial venous sinus with extracranial veins, subserve admirable function of adjusting intracranial pressure.

Splanchno-cranium (visceral cranium), including mandible forms facial skeleton.

Exhibits cavities =

2 orbital

1 nasal

1 oral

(bony palate alveolar processes of upper and lower jaws accommodate teeth bones give attachments to muscles of face which, regulate these apertures.

Facial skeleton develops from visceral (pharyngeal) arches, hence viscorocranium.

CRANIAL CAPACITY

MESOCEPHALIC

SKULL

1350-1450 CM^3

Microcephalic	Megacephalic
< 1350 cm^3	> 1450 cm^3

Approximately 85 named formina, canals and fissures found in skull.

Formina of the base of skull should be identified first.

1. For the entry of internal carotid artery is carotid canal in temporal bone (middle, cranial fossa)
2. For the exit of the jugular vien is jugular foramen in the posterior cranial fossa.
3. The largest foramen, foramen magnum, is in the posterior cranial fossa for the passage of the lowest part of the brain (i) the medulla oblongata (ii) surrounded by meninges (iii) vertebral arteries (1 pair) (iv) internal vertebral plexus of views (v) spinal XI C.N. (vi) apical ligament.

Foramina for the cranial nerves occur in an orderly fashion, for the 1st (olfactory nerve filaments, 12 to 15) in the anterior cranial fossa, through cribiform plate of ethmoid followed from before backwards (restro-caudally) for the 2nd to 12th C.N. in that order

FIGURE

1. Lower end of medulla oblongata.
2. Pia, arachnoid and dura mater
3. Vertebral arteries
4. Internal vertebral plexus of views
5. Spinal accessory C.N.-II nerve ascends
6. Apical ligament

Clinical (applied) Anatomy of skull

1. Bones of calvaria are flat, ossify early in membrane, consist of inner and outer tables of compact bone. In the adult, between 2 tables lies vascular connective tissue (diploi). Diploic views communicate with emissary veins connecting intracranial venous sinuses with extracranial veins.
2. The inner table is thinner, more brittle than the outer. Injury involving outer table, when displaced inwards, may injure the brain. At times, there is no facture in the area of impact but the bone on the opposite side fractures, called contre-coup fracture (French = counter-blow).
3. Periosteum covering outer surface, pericranium, is continuous through sutural ligaments (at the edges of bones, limiting bone) with the inner periosteum, called endocranium sutural ligament between edges of growing bones consists of osteogenic (cambial) and fibrous layers. Ossification in sutural ligaments continues until 30-40 years. The closure of sutures occurs about 10 year earlier on the inner surface.
   In calvaria, sutural closure occurs first in bregma and then extends along sagittal, coronal and bambdoid sutures.
   Premature closure of cranial sutures becomes deformity of skull, craniostenosis.

- If sagittal is suture long and narrow, ridged along closed sagittal suture (this condition is scaphocephaly).
- Premature closure of lamdoid and coronal structures results in sharp pointed head, known as acrophaly (acro = summit, top height)
- Most of bones at base of skull ossify partly in cartilage and partly in membrane. In bones around nasal cavity (para nasal) diploi is replaced by nasal mucous membrane lined air spaces called paranasal air sinuses (thus all communicate with nose). Air in the middle ear (temporal bone) and mastoid process is brought from nasopharynx (via pharyngo-tympanic tube) to maintain an equilibrium of air pressure on both sides of ear drum for proper hearing.

Anatomical position of skull

Orbital cavities are directed horizontally forwards, the lower margin of orbit and upper margin of external acoustic meatus should be in the same horizontal plane (called Frankfurt Plane).

Particular features of individual cranial bones (disarticulated skull) are described separately.

24
Maxilla

Paired, irregular, pneumatic (air filled) bones, both together form upper jaw. Each possesses a pyramidal body and 4 processes.

1. Zyomatic
2. Frontal
3. Alveolar
4. Palatine

BODY

Contains maxillary air sinus (antrum of Highmore), exhibits 4 surfaces

1. Anterior (facial)
2. Posterior (infratemporal)
3. Orbit (floor of orbit) and
4. Nasal or medial,

   large opening of the antrum, the hiatus, seen here.

DETERMINATION OF SIDE

Hold the alveolar border (bearing sockets for teeth) directed downwards; convex surface showing canine eminence and incisive fossa facing forward

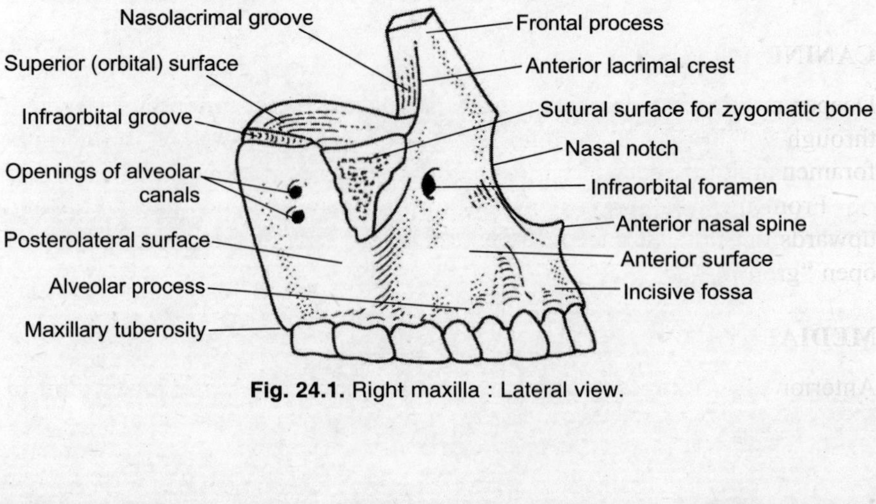

Fig. 24.1. Right maxilla : Lateral view.

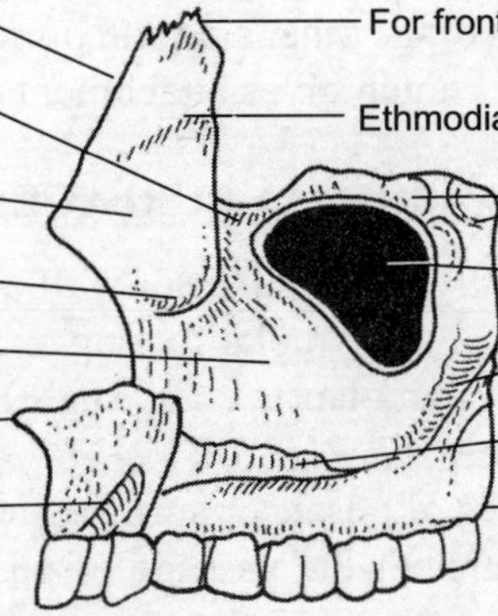

Fig. 24.2. Right maxilla : Medial view.

and laterally, the large surface bearing a hiatus (large opening for antrum) medially with palatal shelf forming its lower limit and the side of maxilla is apparent. One should know at least one each out of 3 pairs of term of position viz. superior/inferior medial/lateral and anterior/posterior, for determining the side of the bone.

PARTICULAR FEATURES OF BODY

Anterior surface: directed forward and laterally. On the anterior surface, close to alveolar border, a linear vertical elevation called canine eminence (caused by the root of canine tooth), is clearly visible. Medial to it, and above the incisor teeth, is a depressed area called incisive fossa. Lateral to canine eminence is located the depression of the canine fossa.

INCISIVE FOSSA

Gives attachment to a part of orbicularis oris (superior incisive band) near alveolar border and depressor septi below nasal aperture. To its upper and lateral part is attached dilator nares.

CANINE FOSSA

Deeper, provides attachment to levator anguli oris below infraorbital foramen, through which exit infraorbital nerve and vessels. Just above infraorbital foramen arises the levator labii superioris.

From the foramen, a bony infraorbital canal extends backwards and upwards to orbital surface of maxilla where it runs further posteriorly as an open "groove".

MEDIALLY

Anterior surface presents a deeply concave nasal notch, the lower limit of which meets a similar notch of the other side and projects forward as "anterior nasal spine" Laterally, nasal notch gives attachment to compressor nares.

POSTERIOR (INFRATEMPORAL) SURFACE

Convex, faces posterolaterally, forms anterior wall of infratemporal fossa. A ridge ascending from the root of 1st molar (acting as a buttress for dispersion of masticatory force from upper molars to cranial base) separates infra-temporal surface from anterior surface.

Three important features of posterior surface are:

1. Foramina near the centre for the passage of posterior superior alveolar nerves and vessels.
2. An oblique groove in upper part, extending laterally and upward, upon which maxillary nerve rests. The groove appears on orbital surface through inferior orbital fissure as one for infraorbital nerve, which infra orbital vessels, accompany.
3. A rounded elevation, maxillary tuberosity, in lower part of this surface, behind the 3rd maxillary molar. It articulates partially with pyramidal process of palatine bone and provides a slip of origin to the superficial head of medial pteygoid.

Orbital Surface

Triangular, forms major part of floor of orbit.

- **Anteriorly:** Limited by lower orbital margin, continuous medially with anterior lacrimal crest of frontal process of maxilla. Free posterior border forms anteromedial boundary of inferior orbital fissure. Near its centre it is marked by the beginning of infraorbital groove, which is continuous anteriorly with infraorbital canal (for infraorbital nerve and vessels). It runs in the roof of maxillary sinus and appears on anterior surface as infraorbital foramen. From the middle of infraorbital canal arises canalis sinuosus, runs at first laterally, then curls medially and downwards below the infraorbital foramen. Anterior superior alveolar nerve and vessels pass through canalis sinuosus.
- Medial margin of orbital surface presents a lacrimal notch in front for the formation of nasolacrimal canal. Rest of the medial margin articulates from before backward with:
  (1) Lacrimal bone
  (2) Orbital plate of ethmoid
  (3) Orbital process of palatine bone

Just lateral to lacrimal notch, the orbital surface gives origin to inferior oblique muscle of eyeball.

NASAL SURFACE OF MAXILLA

The base of maxilla forms the lateral wall of nasal cavity. It presents a large, irregular opening of maxillary sinus, called hiatus. Its upper rough margin articulates with ethmoid labyrinth. Smooth area below hiatus is overlapped by inferior nasal concha. A nasolacrimal groove lies vertically in front of the hiatus, converted into a canal by articulation with descending process of lacrimal bone from above and lacrimal process of inferior concha from below.The maxillary hiatus is narrowed in articulated skull by :

1. Descending process of lacrimal, from above.
2. Maxillary process of inferior concha from below.
3. Uncinate process of ethmoid above and posteriorly.
4. Perpendicular plate of palatine posteriorly ($p\text{-}p\text{-}p\text{-}p = p^4$)

The perpendicular plate of palatine bears a groove which with a sımılar groove on maxilla forms greater palatine canal for the passage of greater palatine nerve and vessels.

ZYGOMATIC PROCESS

Projects laterally from junction of anterior, posterior, orbital surfaces.

It bears a rough triangular area on its upper surface for articulation with maxillary process of zygomatic bone. Represents the apex of pyramidal body of maxilla.

FRONTAL PROCESS

Strong, triangular process, projects upwards with a backward till. Presents a truncated tip.

- 2 borders
  - (i) anterior
  - (ii) posterior
- 2 surfaces
  - (i) medial
  - (ii) lateral

Articulations are as follows:

The tip – with nasal notch of frontal bone.
Anterior border – nasal bone
Posterior border – lacrimal bone

LATERAL SURFACE

Divided by a vertical bony ridge, the anterior lacrimal crest, into anterior and posterior parts. Anterior lacrimal crest gives attachment to lacrimal fascia and near its centre to medial palpebral ligament.Below the ligament it gives attachment to orbicularis oculi, levator labii superioris aleque et nasi, arises further to the front. The posterior part is grooved, with similar groove of adjacent lacrimal bone, it forms lacrimal fossa for lodgement of lacrimal sac.

MEDIAL SURFACE

Marked by a ridge, the ethmoidal crest, sloping downwards and forwards. Posterior part of the crest: articulates with middle nasal concha, anterior free part forms agger nasi. The thick frontal process lies in line of buttress (strengthening) for dispersion of force of impact from anterior teeth to the base of skull.

ALVEOLAR PROCESS

Extends downward and is arched. It is wider posteriorly. It carries sockets for teeth of upper jaw and the alveolar processes of both sides form together the upper alveolar arch. The sockets receive roots of teeth connected by periodontal ligament forming gomphosis (fibrous joint).

- Deepest socket : for canine
- Widest socket : for molars (triple socket for accommodation of 3 roots)

Outer surface of alveolar process opposite the roots of 3 molar teeth gives attachment to buccinator.

Both outer and inner surfaces are covered by mucoperiosteum of gums of upper jaw.

PALATINE PROCESS

Projects medially, as thick horizontal shelf from the junction of nasal surface of body of maxilla and its alveolar process, it articulates with palatine process of opposite maxilla to form the anterior three-fourths of the hard palate. Each process has :

2 surfaces	(i) superior	(ii) inferior
2 borders	(i) medial	(ii) posterior.

INFERIOR SURFACE

Concave, uneven, presents numerous depressions for palatine glands. Postero-laterally, it is marked by 2 grooves for greater palatine vessels and nerves.

The inter-maxillary suture, behind central incisors, involves a conical depression known as incisive fossa. The lateral wall of fossa, on each side, presents an incisive foramen, communicating with floor of nasal cavity. Each incisive foramen transmits long nasopalatine nerve from above and terminal branches of greater palatine arteries from below.

(**Note:** nerves of nasal cavity tend to run beyond it but arteries fall short and arterial reinforcement is received from outside the nasal cavity.)

Sometimes 2 incisive foramina (i) anterior and (ii) posterior, occur. Then, left nasopalatine nerve passes through anterior and right nerve through posterior incisive foramen (left forward – right lags behind, as if marching, left, right, left).

OS INCISIVUM

A suture line, often found to extend bilaterally in young skulls from incisive fossa to junction of lateral incisor and canine teeth. The portion of V-shaped bone in front of the suture is called premaxilla or "os incisivum". Developmentally, from primary palate, it ossified by separate centres.

SUPERIOR SURFACE OF PALATINE PROCESS

Smooth, concave from side to side, forms major part of floor of nasal cavity.

Medial border

articulates with opposite side. Raised nasal crest at the junction, with opposite bone is grooved to receive lower border of vomer. The nasal crest projects anteriorly as "anterior nasal spine."

The posterior, serrated border, articulates with palatine bone.

Ossification

In membrane, a centre above canine fossa in 6th week of intrauterine life. Two centres for premaxilla, in 7th week of embryonic life.

25

The Frontal Bone

THE FRONTAL BONE

The frontal bone is a curved plate of pneumatic flat bone and is shaped like a cockle-shell. It consists of upper, vertical squamous part which forms the forehead, and a pair of horizontal orbital plates which forms the major part of the roof of each orbit. An U-shaped ethmoidal notch intervenes between the orbital plates. (1) Squamous Part - It presents external and internal surfaces, and parietal (posterior) margin. On each side, the supra-orbital margin forms the junction between the squamous part and the orbital plate. The margin is concave, sharp in the lateral two-thirds, and blunt and rounded in the medial one-third. The supraorbital notch or foramen lies at the junction between the two parts of the margin, and transmits supraorbital vessels and nerve; more medially the supra-trochlear vessels and nerve curl upward around the margin.

Traced laterally, the supraorbital margin is continuous with he zygomatic process the tip of which articulates with the frontal process of the zygomatic bone at the frontozygomatic suture. From the posterior margin of each zygomatic process the temporal line curves upwards and backwards, and splits into two lines, superior and inferior temporal, over the parietal bone. The area of external surface of the squamous part below and behind the temporal lines forms the temporal surface on each side, which provides attachment to the temporalis muscle and the overlying temporal fascia.

(2) Between the two supra-orbital margins the squamous part extends downward as the nasal part, which presents a serrated nasal notch at the lower margin. The nasal notch articulates on each side with the nasal bone, frontal process of maxilla and the lacrimal bones. The point of intersection between frontal and nasal bones is known as the nasion. The nasal spine extends downward and forward as a triangular process from the centre of the posterior part of nasal notch. The nasal spine articulates in front with the crest formed by the union of two nasal bones and behind with the perpendicular plate of ethmoid bone. The nasal spine forms a part of nasal septum and is grooved on each side to form the roof of the corresponding part of the nasal cavity.

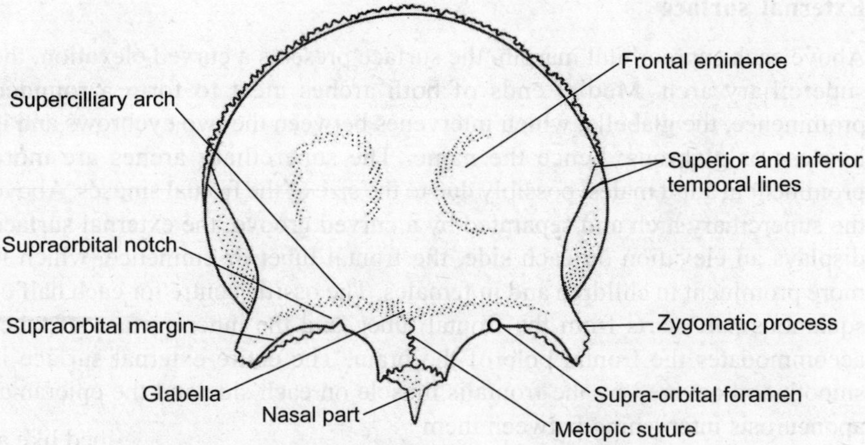

Fig. 25.1. The frontal bone : External surface

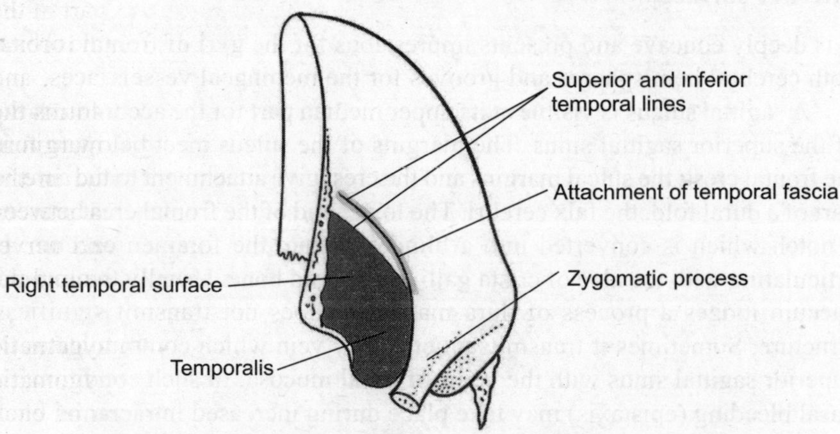

Fig. 25.2. The frontal bone : Right temporal surface in lateral aspect

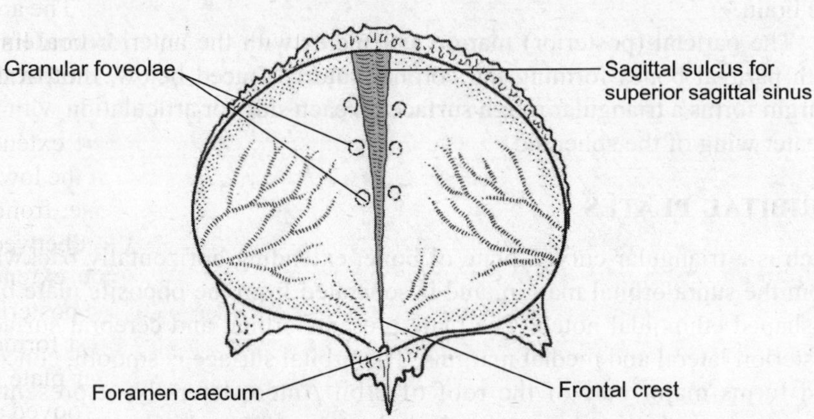

Fig. 25.3. The frontal bone : Internal surface

External surface

Above each supraorbital margin, the surface presents a curved elevation, the superciliary arch. Medial ends of both arches meet to form a rounded prominence, the glabella, which intervenes between the two eyebrows and is hairless or glabrous; hence the name. The superciliary arches are more prominent in adult males, possibly due to the size of the frontal sinuses. Above the superciliary arch and separated by a curved groove, the external surface displays an elevation on each side, the frontal tuber or eminence, which is more prominent in children and in females. The ossific centre for each half of squamous part starts from the frontal tuber, and the inner surface of tuber accommodates the frontal pole of the brain. The entire external surface is smooth and covered by the frontalis muscle on each side and the epicranial aponeurosis intervening between them.

Internal surface

It is deeply concave and presents impressions for the gyri of frontal lobes of both cerebral hemispheres and grooves for the meningeal vessels.

A sagittal sulcus is visible at its upper median part for the accommodation of the superior sagittal sinus. The margins of the sulcus meet below to form the frontal crest; the sulcal margins and the crest give attachment to the anterior part of a dural fold, the falx cerebri. The lower end of the frontal crest presents a notch which is converted into a blind foraman, the foramen caecum, by articulating with the alae of crista galli of ethmoid bone. Usually the foramen caecum lodges a process of dura mater and does not transmit significant structure. Sometimes it transmits an emissary vein which communicates the superior sagittal sinus with the veins of nasal mucosa. In such condition, the nasal bleeding (epistaxis) may take place during increased intracranial blood pressure and acts as a 'safety valve, without producing vascular damage of the brain.

The parietal (posterior) margin articulates with the anterior borders of both parietal bones forming the coronal suture. Traced below, the parietal margin forms a triangular rough surface on each side for articulation with the greater wing of the sphenoid.

ORIBITAL PLATES

Each is a triangular curved plate of bone, extending horizontally backward from the supra orbital margin, and is separated from the opposite plate by a U-shaped ethmoidal notch. The plate presents orbital and cerebral surfaces posterior, lateral and medial margins. The orbital surface is smooth, concave and forms major part of the roof of orbit Antero-laterally, it presents a depression, the lacrimal fossa, for the lodgement of the orbital part of lacrimal gland; the fossa encroaches the zygomatic process of the bone.

Anteromedially, the surface presents a depression or a spine for the attachment of a fibro-cartilaginous pulley through which the superior oblique muscle of eye ball passes and changes direction. The cerebral surface of the orbital plate is convex, irregular and related with the gyri of the orbital surface of frontal lobe. It forms major part of the floor of anterior cranial fossa. The posterior margin articulates with the lesser wing of sphenoid bone. The lateral margin is formed by the triangular rough surface and articulates with the greater wing of sphenoid bone.

The MEDIAL MARGIN is broad and articulates with the upper surface of the labyrinth of ethmoid bone. Two bony canals, anterior and posterior ethmoidal, extend horizontally from the medial wall of the orbit across the area of articulation between the frontal and ethmoid bones, and transmit respectively the anterior and posterior ethmoidal vessels and nerves. The large frontal sinuses, one on each side, are exposed in the anterior part of medial margin. Each frontal sinus is somewhat triangular in outline, extends upward beneath the medial part of superciliary arch at the expense of diploic tissue, and is separated from each other by a bony partition. Each sinus communicates with the middle meatus of the nasal cavity through the frontonasal duct.

The ethmoidal notch intervening between the two orbital plates is occupied by the cribriform plate of ethmoid bone which presents numerous apertures for the passage of olfactory nerves.

OSSIFICATION

Each half of the frontal bone is ossified in membrane from one primary centre which appears near the frontal tuber in the 8th week of intra-uterine life. At birth, the two halves of frontal bone remain separate as the metopic suture, which is replaced by bone at about 2 years. Remnants of the metopic suture may persist in some skulls at the glabella.

At about the 10th year, two secondary centres appear for each half of nasal spine.

26

The Parietal Bone

- **Shape :** Quadrilateral in outline
- **Location :** forms a major portion of the roof and side of the skull
- **Surfaces :** 1. External
  2. Internal
- **Borders :** 1. Superior (sagittal)
  2. Inferior (squamosal)
  3. Anterior (frontal)
  4. Posterior (occipital)
- **Angles:** 1. Antero-superior
  2. Antero-inferior
  3. Postero-superior
  4. Postero-inferior
- **Side determination :**
  1. Antero-inferior angle acute (smallest) grooved on its inner surface by the middle meningeal vessels
  2. External surface is convex

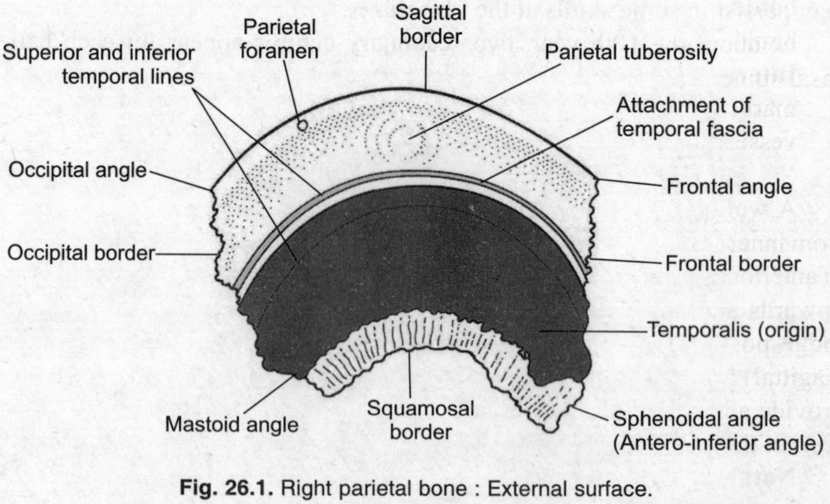

Fig. 26.1. Right parietal bone : External surface.

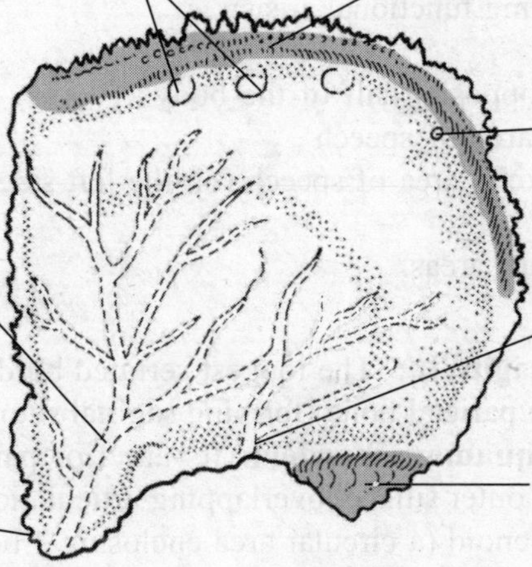

Fig. 26.2. Right parietal bone : Internal surface.

- **External surface :** Convex, smooth, elevated near its centre, called parietal tuber. Two arched lines, superior and inferior temporal lines, with convexity upwards, extend across the bone below the tuber.
- **Attachment :** Superior temporal line
  1. Temporal fascia
  2. Galea aponeurotica, lateral part

  Inferior temporal line and area below, major part of temporal fossa, gives attachment to temporalis muscle. Close to posterior part of superior border, parietal foramen transmits an emissary vein and a meningeal branch from occipital artery.
- **Internal surface :** deeply concave, faces downwards and medially; marked by impressions for cerebral gyri and grooves for meningeal vessels and venous sinuses.

A well defined groove (or bony canal) extends upwards and backwards from inner surface of antero-inferior (sphenoidal) acute angle for the lodgement of anterior division of middle meningeal vessels. Another set of grooves arching upwards and backwards extends from posterior part of inferior border and lodge posterior division of the middle meningeal vessels. Along superior (sagittal) border lies half of a groove for the superior sagittal sinus, margins provide attachment to falx cerebri. Granular pits (for arachnoid granulation) seen in the elderly by the side of the sagittal sulcus.

Notable: The inner surfaces of all 4 angles are related to vessels.

Parietal bone overlaps, partially, all 4 major lobes of cerebral hemisphere and covers the following functional areas:

1. Motor area
2. Sensory area of opposite half of the body
3. Motor (Broca's) area of speech
4. Sensory (Wernicke's) area of speech (on the left side in right handers).
5. Primary and
6. Secondary auditory areas.

- **Borders**
  1. **Superior (sagittal) :** The longest serrated border articulates with the opposite parietal bone (forming sagittal suture)
  2. **Inferior (squamous border):** Its anterior part projects below, bevelled on outer suface, overlapping articulation with the greater wing of sphenoid (a circular area enclosing 4 bones, viz. parietal, greater wing of sphenoid bone, squamous temporal and frontal known as pterion)

     Posterior part : articulates with the upper border of mastoid part of temporal bone.
  3. **Anterior border (frontal):** is serrated bevelled on outer surface in upper part, on inner surface in lower part. Articulates with squamous frontal bone, forms half of coronal suture.
  4. **Posterior (occipital) border :** dentale articulates with the occipital bone, forms half of lambdoid suture.

- **Particular features of angles**
  1. **Anterosuperior (frontal):** makes a right angle bend, forms bregma (formed after the fusion of the anterior frontanelle at 1 ½ to 2 years of age) at the meeting point of the coronal and sagittal suture.
  2. **Posterosuperior (occipital) angle:** meeting point of sagittal and lambdoid sutures, forms lambda.
  3. **Antero-inferior (sphenoidal) angle:** juts downwards, a meeting place of 4 bones separated by H-shaped sutures:
     (a) Squamous frontal bone
     (b) Greater wing of sphenoid bone
     (c) Squamous part temporal bone
     (d) Antero-inferior angle of the parietal bone

Region occupied by H-shaped suture (enclosing the 4 bones) is known as the pterion, deep to which lies anterior division of the middle meningeal vessels.

OSSIFICATION

Ossification : intramembranous 2 primary centres, one above the other appears at the parietal tube in the 7th week of the intrauterine life. Both fuse easily and ossification spreads centrifugally to borders first and angles later. Unossified membranous gaps at the 4 angles form the frontanelles (for details see norma verticalis in neonatal skull on page 14).

APPLIED ANATOMY

Middle meningeal vessels running in the bony groove of antero-inferior angle commonly bleed in head injuries (road accidents) and epidural or extradural haematoma results. Classical presentation is unconsciousness (due to concussion of brain) soon after head injury, then a lucid (clear) interval, when the patient regains consciousness and thereafter loses consciousness again due to compression of the brain by the resultant extradural haematoma. It is a surgical emergency and needs immediate craniotomy and removal of blood clot.

27

The Palatine Bone

Paired palatine bones intervene between the maxillae in front and the pterygoid processes of sphenoid behind. Each bone is L shaped and consists of horizontal and perpendicular plates, and three processes:

1. Orbital
2. Sphenoidal
3. Pyramidal

HORIZONTAL PLATE

quadrilateral in shape and presents 2 surfaces, nasal and palatine, and four borders – anterior, posterior, lateral and medial.

The nasal surface is concave from side to side and forms the posterior part of the floor of nasal cavity.

The anterior border articulates with the palatine process of maxilla.

The posterior border is free and concave and presents medially a conical backward projection which with its fellow forms the posterior nasal spine. The expanded tendon of tensor veli palatine (palatine aponeurosis) is attached along the posterior border and extends upto the palatine crest; the posterior nasal spine gives attachment to musculus uvulae.

The lateral border is continuous with the perpendicular plate. It is marked by the lower end of the greater palatine groove.

The medial border articulates with its fellow and forms a raised nasal crest which joins with the lower border of the vomer.

Perpendicular plate

It is an oblong, vertical plate, and possesses two surfaces, nasal and maxillary, and four borders:

1. Anterior,
2. Posterior
3. Superior
4. Inferior

The nasal surface forms the lateral wall of the nasal cavity, just in front of the medial pterygoid plate. It is marked by two horizontal bony ridges, the conchal crest below and the ethmoidal crest above. The conchal crest articulates with the inferior nasal concha and the area below it is depressed to form the lateral orbital process wall of the inferior meatus.

The ethmoidal crest articulates with the middle nasal concha and the depressed area between the ethmoidal and conchal crests forms the lateral wall of the middle meatus. Further above the bethmoidal crest there lies a narrow groove for the superior meatus.

The maxillary (lateral) surface presents 3 parts:

1. Intermediate
2. Postero-superior
3. Antero-inferior

The intermediate and major part articulate with the nasal surface of the body of maxilla behind the maxillary hiatus and bears an oblique deep groove which, with the similar groove of maxilla, forms a bony canal for the transmission of greater palatine vessels and nerves.

The postero-superior part is smooth and forms the medial wall of pterygo-palatine fossa. The antero-inferior part is also smooth, overlaps the posterior part of maxillary hiatus and forms the medial wall of the maxillary sinus.

The anterior border projects forward in the lower part as the maxillary process overlaps the maxillary hiatus and articulates with the similar process of inferior nasal concha.

The posterior border articulates with the medial pterygoid plate. It is continuous above with the sphenoid process and below with the pyramidal process of palatine bone (see later).

The superior border carries the orbital process in front and sphenoidal process behind, separated by the sphenopalatine notch; the latter is converted by the body of the sphenoid into into a sphenopalatine foramen, which communicates the pterygo-palatine fossa with the posterior part of superior meatus and transmits sphenopalatine vessels and posterior superior nasal nerves. The orbital process lies at a higher level and diverges above. Whereas the sphenoidal process converges above.

The inferior border is continuous with the lateral border of the horizontal plate.

Pyramidal Process: It projects postero-laterally from the junction of the perpendicular and horizontal plates and articulate with the margins of the pterygoid fissure between the two pterygoid plates. The pyramidal process presents posterior, lateral and inferior surfaces.

The posterior surface forms a part of floor of pterygoid fossa and gives attachment to the medial pterygoid muscle. The lateral surface articulates in front with the maxillary tuberosity, and the rest forms the medial wall of the infratemporal fossa. The inferior surface presents foramina for the lesser palatiné vessels and nerves.

ORBITAL PROCESS

It projects upward and laterally as an expanded process from the superior border of the perpendicular plate and in front of the sphenopalatine notch. It contains an air sinus and presents five surfaces – 3 articular and 2 non-articular.

The articular surfaces are:

1. Maxillary, directed antero-laterally and joins with the body of maxilla.
2. Ethmoidal, directed antero-medially and articulates with the labyrinth of ethmoid.
3. Sphenoidal, directed postero-medially with an upward tilt and articulates with the sphenoidal concha. It usually bears an opening for the air sinus and communicates with the sphenoidal sinus.

The non-articular surfaces are:

1. Orbital or superior surface which is triangular and forms the most posterior part of the floor of the orbit.
2. Lateral surface, forming the medial wall of pterygo-palatine fossa is separated from the orbital surface by a rounded border; the latter forms the medial part of lower border of the inferior orbital fissue.

SPHENOIDAL PROCESS

It projects upward and medially from the superior border of perpendicular plate and behind the sphenopalatine notch. It presents 3 surfaces and 3 borders.

The superior surface is articular and joins with the sphenoidal concha; further behind it carries a groove and is overlapped by the vaginal process of medial pterygoid to form the palatino-vaginal (pharyngeal) canal (see the sphenoid bone). The inferomedial surface is concave and forms the roof and lateral wall of the nasal cavity. The lateral surface forms the medial wall of pterygopalatinefossa.

The anterior border forms the spheno-palatine (vide supra). The posterior border articulates with the vaginal process of medial pterygoid plate. The medial border articulates with the lateral margin of the ala of the vomer.

OSSIFICATION

Each bone is ossified in membrane from one centre which appears in the perpendicular plate in the 8th intra-uterine week.

28
Interior of the Skull

The interior of the skull may be divided into two regions—inner surface of the calvaria, and the interior of the base of skull.

INNER SURFACE OF THE CALVARIA

It shows the coronal, sagittal and lambdoid sutures. The surface is grooved in the midline by the sagittal sulcus which becomes deeper as it is traced behind to the internal occipital protuberance, where the sulcus is continuous with the right or left transverse sulcus. The sagittal sulcus lodges the superior sagittal sinus.The frontal crest anteriorly and the lips of sagittal sulcus provide attachment to a sickle-shaped fold of dura mater, the falx cerebri.

A number of irregular depressions known as granular pits are found on each side of the sagittal sulcus. Lacunae and arachnoid granulations which help absorption of cerebrospinal fluid into the venous sinuses.

Numerous grooves affect the calvaria for meningeal vessels. The largest are on the parietal bones for the branches of middle meningeal vessels. The terminal branches of middle meningeal artery are separated from the bone by their corresponding veins. Therefore the vascular grooves are produced mostly by the veins rather than the arter!es.

One or more parietal foramina open on this surface close to the sagittal groove about 3.5 cm in front of lambdoid suture. The foramen transmits emissary vein communicating with the superior sagittal sinus.

INTERIOR OF THE BASE OF THE SKULL

Base of the skull is divisible into three terraces or descending steps - anterior, middle and posterior cranial fossae

The anterior and middle fossae are separated from each other by the posterior border of the lesser wing of the sphenoid on each side, and the anterior border of the sulcus chiasmaticus in the median region.

The middle cranial fossa is marked off from the posterior fossa by the upper border of petrous temporal on each side, and dorsum sellae of sphenoid bone in the middle.

ANTERIOR CRANIAL FOSSA: It lodges the frontal lobes of the brain, and is floored by portions of three bones—cribriform plate of the ethmoid, orbital plates of the frontal, and lesser wings with jugum sphenoidale of the sphenoid.

The cribriform plate of the ethmoid forms the roof of nasal cavity. On each side it presents a number of small apertures for the passage of olfactory nerves from the nasal mucosa to the olfactory bulbs. Posteriorly it articulates with the jugum sphenoidale of the body of sphenoid that roofs the sphenoidal air sinus. A median triangular process, the crista galli, projects upward from the cribriform plate. The crista along with the frontal crest gives attachment to the falx cerebri. A foramen caecum with a blind lower end intervenes between the crista and the frontal crest; rarely it transmits a vein from the nasal mucosa to the superior sagittal sinus.

Medial ends of anterior and posterior ethmoidal canals open extradurally on each side of the cribriform plate. They transmit respectively anterior and posterior ethmoidal vessels and nerves from the orbital cavity. Anterior ethmoidal vessels and nerve extend further into the nasal cavity through a slit-like aperture by the side of crista galli.

Each **orbital plate** of frontal bone is convex, and forms the roof of the orbit and ethmoidal sinuses. It articulates behind with the lesser wing of the sphenoid.

Each **lesser wing** presents a concave, sharp posterior margin (sphenoidal ridge) which overhangs the middle cranial fossa and projects into the lateral sulcus of cerebral hemisphere. The medial end of posterior margin forms a projecting tubercle, the anterior clinoid process, which gives attachment to the anterior end of the free margin of tentorium cere belli.

MIDDLE CRANIAL FOSSA: It contains hypophysis cerebri in the middle and temporal lobe of the brain on each side. The floor of the fossa, is shaped like a butterfly, and consists of a small median part and a pair of expanded lateral parts.

Median part: It is formed by the upper surface of the body of sphenoid, and presents the sulcus chiasmaticus in front, sella turcica behind, and carotid groove on each side.

The sulcus chiasmaticus is a shallow transverse groove which leads on each side to the optic canal. The optic chiasma does not lodge in the sulcus, but lies slightly above it. Each optic canal is directed toward and laterally to open into the orbit, and is bounded by the two roots of lesser wing and the body of sphenoid. The canal transmits the optic nerve accompanied infero-laterally by the ophthalmic artery.

The **sella turcica** resembles a Turkish saddle and consists of tuberculum sellae, hypophyseal fossa and dorsum sellae from before backward..

The hypophyseal fossa is a deep depression, which contains hypophysis cerebri or pituitary gland. The floor of the fossa is related to the sphenoidal air sinus.

Dorsum sellae is a square-like plate of bone which projects upward and presents a posterior clinoid process on each side. The posterior clinoid process gives attachment to the anterior and of the attached margin of tentorium cerebelli. Just by the side, of the clinoid process, the free and attached margins of tentorium cerebelli cross each other and the triangular area of the meningeal layer of dura mater in front of the crossing is pierced by the oculomotor and trochlear nerves; hence this area is sometimes called the oculomotor trigone. Below the posterior clinoid process; the lateral margin of dorsum sellae presents a petrosal process which is connected to the tip of petrous temporal by a petrosphenoid ligament; immediately below that ligament the abducent nerve pierces the dura mater and appears in the cavernous sinus through the osseo-ligamentous foramen after forming an angular bend.

An italic 'f' shaped **carotid groove** is seen on each side of sella turcica. It lodges the internal carotid artery surrounded by a plexus of sympathetic nerves. The carotid artery passes at first upward through the upper opening of foramen lacerum, then forward along the groove and finally turns upward medial to the anterior clinoid process. Posteriorly the groove is deepened on the lateral side by a triangular projection, the lingula.

Each lateral part of the middle cranial fossa is formed by the cranial surface of the greater wing of the sphenoid, inner surface of squamous part and anterior surface of petrous part of the temporal.

(1) The greater wing is deeply concave and presents along a crescentic line the following foramina before backward—superior orbital fissure, foramen rotundum, foramen ovale, and foramen spinosum.

The **superior orbital fissure** is an oblique cleft and communicates with the orbit. The fissure is bounded above and medially by the lower surface of the lesser wing, below and laterally by the medial margin of the orbital surface of greater wing, and medially by the body of sphenoid. The fissure is subdivided by the attachment of common tendinous ring (for the origin of four recti muscles of eyeball) into three parts—lateral, intermediate and medial. The lateral part transmits lacrimal, frontal and trochlear nerves, lacrimal branch of middle meningeal and recurrent meningeal branch of ophthalmic arteries, and superior ophthalmic vein or veins. The intermediate part (within the tendinous ring) transmits superior and inferior rami of oculomotor nerve, nasociliary and abducent nerves, and occasionally superior ophthalmic veins. The medial part transmits inferior ophthalmic veins.

The **foramen rotundum** lies immediately behind the medial end of superior orbital fissure. It forms a round bony canal, and transmits the maxillary nerve from the trigeminal ganglion to the pterygopalatine fossa.

The **foramen ovale** is located behind and lateral to foramen rotundum, and opens into the roof of infratemporal fossa. It transmits mandibular nerve from the trigeminal ganglion.

The foramen spinosum: It transmits the entrance of middle meningeal artery and nervous spinosus.

(2) The inner surface of squamous temporal presents a groove for middle meningeal artery, which curves forward and laterally from the foramen spinosum to a point corresponding to the middle of the zygomatic arch. The groove divides here into two for the anterior and posterior branches of middle meningeal artery. The anterior groove proceeds to the inner aspect of pterion as an open groove or a bony canal and finally ascends to the vertex. The posterior groove curves backward above and parallel to the zygomatic arch and supramastoid crest.

(3) The anterior surface of the petrous temporal presents the following features;

   (a) Trigeminal impression forms a shallow fossa close to the apex of petrous part and postero-lateral to foramen lacerum. It lodges the trigeminal ganglion in a pouch of dura mater, the cavum trigeminale. The impression is continuous behind with a notch that affects the medial part of upper border of petrous bone for the lodgement of sensory and motor roots of trigeminal nerve.

   (b) Arcuate eminence overlies the anterior semicircular canal of the internal ear.

   (c) Tegmen tympani is a thin plate of bone which covers rest of the anterior surface of petrous part. It forms a common roof from behind forward of mastoid antrum, tympanic cavity and bony part of auditory tube. Lateral part of tegmen tympani projects downward to divide the squamotympanic fissure into two parts.

   The tegmen tympani presents two foramina, lateral and medial, from each of which a faint groove runs antero-medially. The lateral foramen transmits lesser petrosal nerve (from glossopharyngeal): the medial foramen transmits greater petrosal nerve (from facial).

(4) Foramen lacerum - *(see* norma basalis).

POSTERIOR CRANIAL FOSSA

It is the deepest of the three fossae and lodges the hindbrain consisting of cerebellum, pons and medulla oblongata.

In life the roof of the posterior fossa is formed by a dural fold, the tentorium cerebelli, which intervenes between the occipital lobes of cerebral hemispheres above and the cerebellum below. The tentorium is attached to the upper borders of petrous temporal and the lips of the transverse sulci on the inner surface of the occipital.

The floor of the posterior fossa presents a large oval-shaped central opening, the foramen magnum, which is described in norma basalis. The bones forming the floor are sphenoid, occipital, temporal and postero-inferior angles of the parietal.

In front of foramen magnum, a sloping surface of bone known as the clivus ascends to the dorsum sellae, and is formed by the fusion of the basi-occiput and the body of the sphenoid. The clivus is related to the pons and medulla oblongata, separated by the basilar artery with its branches and basilar venous plexus. The inferior petrosal sinus lies in the groove between the basilar part and petrous temporal. Close to the anterior margin of foramen magnum, the basilar part gives attachment from above downward to the membrana tectoria, upper band of cruciate ligament and apical ligament.

Behind the foramen magnum, the inner surface of the occipital bone presents a median ridge, the internal occipital crest, which extends upward upto the internal occipital protuberance. The falx cerebelli is attached to the crest and intervenes between the two cerebellar hemispheres. The internal crest diverges below to form a triangular depression, the vermian fossa, which lodges the inferior vermis of cerebellum. A transverse sulcus extends laterally from each side of internal occipital protuberance. The transverse sulci lodge right and left transverse sinuses and the lips of the sulci give attachment to the tentorium cerebelli. Traced further laterally each transverse sulcus curves downward as sigmoid sulcus which involves the inner surface of the postero-inferior angle of parietal, mastoid part of temporal and upper surface. of jugular process of occipital bone. The sigmoid sulcus lodges sigmoid sinus which leaves the skull through the posterior compartment of jugular foramen as the internal jugular vein. The sigmoid sinus is related to the posterior wall of mastoid antrum separated by mastoid air cells. Two emissary veins communicate with sigmoid sinus - one through the mastoid canal in close proximity to the occipito-mastoid suture, and the other (occasional) through the posterior condylar canal.

The Internal occipital protuberance is the meeting place of falx cerebri, falx cerebelli and the tentorium cerebelli. Here is a confluence of venous sinuses (torcula Hirophili), where superior sagittal sinus is usually continuous with the right transverse sinus and straight sinus with left transverse sinus; the arrangement of confluence of sinuses is, however, variable.

On each side of foramen magnum, the following features are seen;

- **Hypoglossal canal** - It lies a little above the anterior part of lateral margin of foramen magnum, and transmits hypoglossal nerve and the accompanying vessels (*see* norma basalis).

- Tuberculum jugulare is an elevation above the hypoglossal canal and projects into the postero-medial boundary of jugular foramen. The tubercle is crossed by the oblique grooves for the passage of glossopharyngeal, vagus and accessory nerves from before backward.
  - Jugular foramen: Boundaries and structures passing through the foramen are described in norma basalis.

Posterior surface of the petrous temporal is triangular. Its three borders are accompanied by venous sinuses - superior border by superior petrosal sinus, posterior border by sigmoid sinus, and antero-inferior border by inferior petrosal sinus. The posterior surface displays the following features;

- Internal acoustic meatus ia a bony canal, about 1 cm. long, and lies in line with the external acoustic meatus. It transmits the facial and vestibulo-cochlear nerves, and labyrinthine artery. Lateral end of the internal meatus is closed by a bony plate which is subdivided by a horizontal crest into upper and lower parts. The upper part presents- the opening of facial canal in front, superior vestibular area behind for the passage of upper division of vestibular nerve. The lower part presents tractus splralls foramlnosus in front for cochlear nerve, Inferior vestibular area behind for lower division of vestibular nerve. A foramen slngulare lies behind and below the inferior vestibular area.
- The subarcuate fossa is an indistinst depression situated behind and lateral to the internal meatus. It lodges a process of dura mater and transmits some blood vessels. The subarcuate fossa is prominent in the new born.
- Behind the internal meatus there lies an oblique slit which leads upward to a bony canal, the aqueduct of vestibule. It lodges saccus and ductus endolymphaticus.
- Just above the anterior end of jugular foramen, the lower border of petrous part presents a pyramidal notch which lodges the inferior ganglion of glossopharyngeal nerve. From the apex of pyramid a tiny cochlear canal lodges the aqueduct of cochlea.

Note: A coronal plane drawn downward through the internal acoustic meatus is related to the last six cranial nerves: 7th and 8th nerves in the internal acoustic meatus; 9th, 10th and 11th nerves in the jugular foramen; 12th nerve in the hypoglossal canal.

POINTS TO REMEMBER (SUMMARY)

Passage of cranial nerves through the base of skull: The cranial nerves pass in numerical order from anterior to posterior as follows.

- First cranial or olfactory nerves (15 to 20 fasciculi on each side)- through the cribriform plate of the ethmoid and join with the olfactory bulbs.
- Second cranial or optic nerve-through the optic canal and joins with optic chiasma.
- Third cranial or oculomotor nerve-through the intermediate compartment of superior orbital fissure by dividing into superior and inferior rami.
- Fourth cranial or trochlear nerve-through the lateral compartment of superior orbital fissure.
- Fifth cranial or trigeminal nerve
  - Ophthalmic division (V1) divides into three branches-lacrimal, frontal and nasociliary.

    Lacrimal and frontal branches - through the lateral compartment of superior orbital fissure. Nasociliary-through the intermediate compartment of superior orbital fissure.
  - Maxillary division (V2) - through the foramen rotundum.
  - Mandibular division (V3) - through the foramen ovale.
- Sixth cranial or abducent nerve - through the intermediate compartment of superior orbital fissure.
- Seventh cranial or facial nerve-through the internal acoustic meatus and leaves the exterior of skull through the stylomastoid foramen.
- Eighth cranial or vestibulo-cochlear nerve-from the internal ear through the internal acoustic meatus.
- Ninth, tenth and eleventh cranial nerves (glossopharyngeal, vagus and accessory nerves-through the intermediate compartment of jugular foramen.
- Twelfth cranial or hypoglossal nerve-through the hypoglossal canal of occipital bone.

29

Norma Basalis

ANTERIOR PART

It comprises the bony palate and alveolar arch.

Bony palate

It lies within the alveolar arch and is slightly arched from before backwards and from side to side. The bony palate is formed by the assembly of the palatine processes of maxillae and horizontal parts of palatine bones, separated by a cruciform suture. Bony palate 3/4th is contributed by maxillae and 1/4th by the palatine bones. Posteriorly, it ends in a crescentic free margin which presents a midline backward projection, the posterior nasal spine; the latter

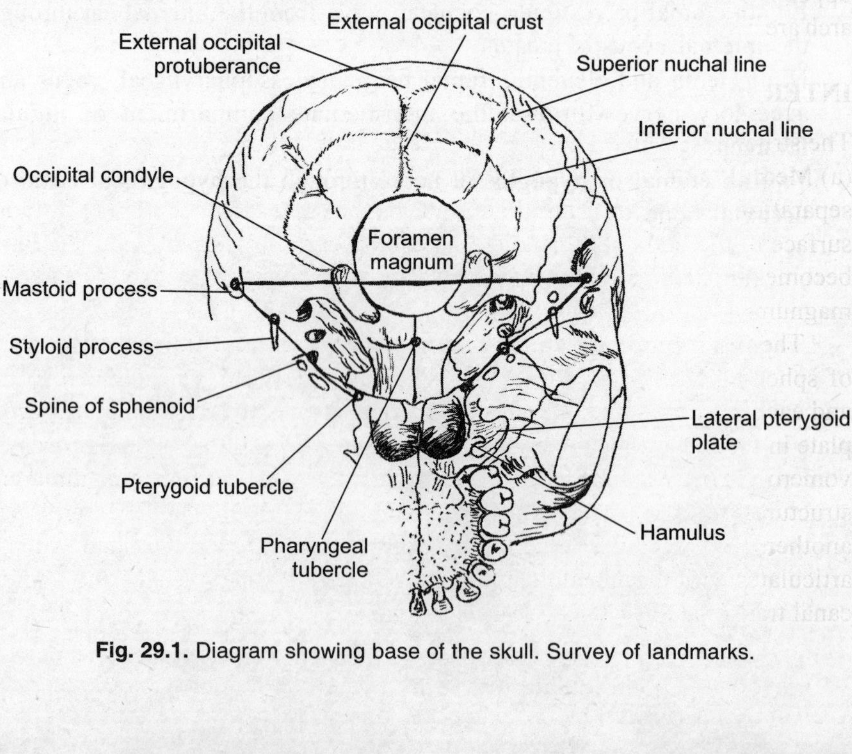

Fig. 29.1. Diagram showing base of the skull. Survey of landmarks.

gives attachment to musculus uvulae on each side. The free margin of hard palate extending upto the palatine crest provides the insertion of tensor veli palatini in the form of palatine aponeurosis.

The **greater palatine foramen** is situated close to the lateral border of hard palate medial to the third molar tooth. The foramen transmits greater palatine vessels and nerves. The **lesser palatine foramina:** usually two on each side, lie just behind the greater palatine foramen in the pyramidal process of palatine bone which is wedged between the lower ends of medial and lateral pterygoid plates of the sphenoid. The lesser foramina convey corresponding vessels and nerves.

The incisive fossa, a conical depression, involves the intermaxillary suture behind the central incisor teeth. The lateral wall of the fossa presents on each side lateral incisive foramen which communicates with the floor of the nasal cavity. Each foramen transmits long naso-palatine nerve from above and terminal branches of greater palatine vessels from below. Sometimes anterior and posterior incisive foramina affect the anterior and posterior walls of the fossa respectively. When present, the anterior foramen transmits left long nasopalatine nerve and the posterior foramen right long nasopalatine nerve. On occasions, a sutural line is found to extend bilaterally in young skulls from the incisive fossa to the junction between lateral incisor and canine teeth. The portion of the bone in front of the suture is known as pre-maxilla which is ossified from separate centres.

Alveolar arch: is horse-shoe shaped and provides sockets for the teeth of upper jaw. Posterior to the third molars, buccal and lingual surfaces of the arch are continuous, and above that continuity the maxilla presents a tuberosity.

INTERMEDIATE PART

The structures are subdivided into median and para-median parts.

(a) Median structures from before backwards are: posterior border of vomer separating the posterior nasal apertures or choanae from each other, inferior surface of the body of sphenoid, and basilar part of occipital bone; the latter becomes broader as it slopes downward and backward to reach the foramen magnum.

The upper border of vomer diverges into two alae as it reaches the body of sphenoid. The grooved margin articulates with the sphenoidal rostrum, and each ala meets and overlaps the vaginal process of the medial pterygoid plate in the interval between the body of sphenoid and the vaginal process; a vomero-vaginal canal between them runs forward without containing important structures. Inferior surface of the vaginal process presents in the anterior part another groove which is converted into a palatino-vaginal canal when it articulates with the sphenoidal process of palatine bone; the palatino-vaginal canal transmits pharyngeal vessels and nerve.

Intermediate area presents from before backward

- Medial and lateral pterygoid plates extending downward behind the third molar tooth and lateral to the choana;
- the infra-temporal surface of the greater wing of the sphenoid spreading horizontally lateralward from the root of the lateral pterygoid plate;
- squamous, tympanic and petrous parts of temporal bone:
  - The posterior border of medial pterygoid plate is free. Traced above, it forms the scaphoid fossa for the principal attachment of tensor veli palatini, and further above it leads to a tubercle which overlaps the posterior opening of the pterygoid canal in the anterior wall of foramen lacerum. Traced below, the posterior border projects downward and laterally as a hook-like projection, the hamulus, around which the tendon of tensor veli palatini turns medially to enter the soft palate. The middle of the posterior which supports the medial end of the cartilagenous part of auditory tube. Rest of the border below the processus gives attachment to the pharyngo, basilar fascia and superior constrictor muscle. Pterygoid hamulus is connected to the mandible behind the third molar tooth by the pterygomandibular raphe.

    The lateral pterygoid plate is called "the muscular plate." Its medial surface gives origin to the medial pterygoid muscle. Its lateral gives origin to the lower head of lateral pterygoid muscle. A bony process is connected to the spine of sphenoid bone by the pterygo-spinous ligament.
  - Infratemporal surface of the greater wing of sphenoid forms the roof of infratemporal fossa. It is roughly pentagonal; the anterior margin forms the postero lateral boundary of inferior orbital fissure, and antero laterally limited by the infratemporal crest. Laterally it articulates with the squamous temporal and medially it is continuous with the root of lateral pterygoid plate. Its postero-medial border articulates with the petrous temporal and a sulcus tubae formed between them lodges the cartilagenous part of auditory tube.

    This surface gives origin to the upper head of lateral pterygoid muscle, and presents foramen ovale, foramen spinosum and spine of the sphenoid.

    The foramen ovale transmits:

1. two roots of mandibular nerve (motor and sensory),
2. accessory meningeal artery, occasionally,
3. lesser petrosal nerve
4. an emissary vein communicating cavernous sinus with pterygoid venous plexus, and
5. anterior division of middle meningeal sinus.

The foramen spinosum lies postero-lateral to foramen ovale. It transmits:

1. middle meningeal artery,
2. nervous spinosus from the trunk of mandibular nerve.

Postero lateral to the foramen spinosum, the greater wing presents a triangular downward projection, the spine of the sphenoid. The spine provides attachments to 2 muscles:

1. the tensor veli palatini,
2. tensor tympani, and

3 ligaments:

1. spheno-mandibular,
2. pterygo-spinous,
3. anterior ligament of malleus. The spine is related laterally to the auriculo-temporal nerve, and medially to the chorda tympani nerve and the auditory tube as it lodges in the sulcus tubae.

– The zygomatic process of squamous temporal presents a tubercle, where it separates into anterior and posterior roots enclosing between them the anterior part of mandibular fossa. The anterior root forms the articular eminence.

The mandibular fossa presents an anterior articular part formed by squamous temporal, and a posterior non-articular part formed by the anterior surface of tympanic plate of temporal bone. The articular part including articular eminence, receives the head of the mandible separated by an articular disc and enters the formation of temporo-mandibular joint. The non-articular part of the fossa is separated from the joint by a portion of parotid gland.

A squamo-tympanic fissure intervenes between the articular and non-articular parts of the fossa. The down turned edge of tegmen tympani of petrous temporal encroaches the medial part of the fissure, and divides the latter into petro-squamous fissure in front and petro-tympanic fissure behind.

The petro-tympanic fissure transmits at its medial end:

1. the chorda tympanic nerve,
2. anterior tympanic branch of maxillary artery and
3. anterior ligament of malleus.

The lateral border of the tympanic plate forms the antero-inferior margin on the outer opening of external acoustic meatus. The lower border of tympanic plate is sharp and incorporated with the inferior surface of petrous temporal; here it splits to enclose the root of the styloid process of temporal and acts as a sheath for the styloid process.

The inferior surface of the petrous temporal intervenes between the greater wing of the sphenoid and the basilar part of the occipital bones. The apex of the petrous part is separated from the body of the sphenoid by a bony canal with irregular margin, the foramen lacerum. The foramen (is not in a single bone): is bounded in front by the body and the greater wing of sphenoid bone.

The foramen magnum is oval in outline, wider behind than in front, and communicates the posterior cranial fossa with the vertebral canal. The foramen is located midway between and on a level with the mastoid processes. On each side of the foramen, a tubercle of the occipital condyle projects slightly medially and gives attachment to the alar ligament from the dens. The foramen magnum is divided by the alar ligaments into anterior small and posterior large compartments.The most important structure passing through this largest foramen of cranium (containing brain) is the lower end of brainstem, the medulla oblongata.

Details of structures passing through the anterior compartment are from before backward:

1. apical ligament,
2. upper band of cruciate ligament, and
3. membrana tectoria.

Therefore, the anterior compartment of the foramen may be called the osseo-ligamentous compartment. Structures passing through the posterior compartment are the following: the lower end of medulla oblongata and the meninges, fourth part of vertebral arteries surrounded by sympathetic plexus of nerves, spinal roots of accessory nerves, anterior and posterior spinal arteries, and occasionally tonsils of the cerebellum projecting on each side of the brain stem. Therefore the posterior compartment may be called the neuro-vascular compartment. The anterior and posterior margins of foramen magnum give attachment respectively to anterior and posterior atlanto-occipital membranes. The middle point of anterior margin of foramen magnum is known as the basion.

The squamous part of occipital bone presents in the mid line an external occipital crest, extending from the foramen magnum to the external occipital protuberance. The crest and protuberance give attachment to the upper end of ligamentum nuchae. The arched superior nuchal lines extend bilaterally from external protuberance *(see* norma verticalis). From the middle of the external occipital crest the inferior nuchal lines extend bilaterally parallel to the superior nuchal lines. The area of occipital bone between the superior and inferior nuchal lines gives attachment on each side to the semispinalis capitis medially, and obliquus capitis superior laterally. The area between the inferior nuchal line and posterior margin of foramen magnum receives attachment of rectus capitis posterior minor medially, the rectus capitis posterior major laterally.

The condylar parts of occipital bone consist of:

1. occipital condyles, and
2. jugular processes.

The occipital condyle is set obliquely so that the anterior end is nearer to the median plane. The articular surface is convex and articulates with the upper surface of the lateral mass of atlas. The junction between the basilar and condylar parts is represented by a line across the anterior one-thirds and posterior two-third of the condyle. Above the anterior part of the condyle the hypoglossal (anterior condylar) canal extends forward and laterally, and transmits the hypoglossal nerve, meningeal branch of ascending pharyngeal artery and occasionally an emissary vein. A condylar fossa is present behind each condyle for accommodation of posterior margin of the lateral mass of atlas during backward nodding of the head. Sometimes posterior condylar foramen is present; it transmits an emissary vein connecting sigmoid sinus with sub-occipital venous plexus, and occasionally a meningeal branch of occipital artery.

Each jugular process articulates laterally with the petrous temporal by a primary cartilagenous joint, and its inferior surface is rough for the attachment of rectus capitis lateralls muscle. The anterior margin of jugular process is free and is called the jugular notch which forms the posterior boundary of jugular foramen.

The jugular foramen is a large irregular opening, the long axis being directed forward and medially.The anterior part transmits inferior petrosal sinus (first tributary of internal jugular vein), middle part gives passage to the glosso-pharyngeal, vagus and accessory nerves with meningeal branch of ascending pharyngeal artery and occasional emissary veins, and the posterior part conveys internal jugular vein as a continuation of sigmoid sinus. The commencement of internal jugular vein presents a dilatation, the superior bulb, which lodges in the jugular fossa of petrous temporal. Lateral wall of the fossa presents one or more mastoid canaliculi for the auricular branch of vagus nerve. Just in front of the fossa lies lower opening of the carotid canal, separated by a bony ridge which presents tympanic canaliculus for the tympanic branch of glossopharyngeal nerve. In front of jugular fossa and medial to the carotid canal lies a triangular depression for the lodgement of inferior ganglion of glossopharyngeal nerve; from the apex of the depression a cochlear canaliculus extends upward and transmits aqueduct of cochlea which communicates the perilymph with the cerebro-spinal fluid of the subarachnoid space.

Lateral to the jugular fossa the styloid process of temporal bone emerges from its sheath and projects downward and forward for a variable distance. Postero-lateral to the styloid process the mastoid process presents a conical projection with notch on its medial surface for the origin of the posterior belly of digastric muscle. Medial to the digastric notch a groove runs backward and upward for the lodgement of occipital artery.

The **stylomastoid foramen,** appears midway between the styloid and mastoid processes. It transmits the facial nerve and stylomastoid artery.

Datum lines: Three transverse datum lines—posterior, middle and anterior, are found useful to consider some of the features at the base of the skull.

Posterior transverse line passes through the posterior border of external acoustic meatus, and the following structures lie along the line:

1. stylomastoid foramen,
2. posterior margin of jugular foramen,
3. hypoglossal canal, and
4. junction between the anterior one-third and posterior two-thirds of occipital condyle.

Middle transverse line passes through the mandibular fossa and the following structures are encountered along it:

1. petrotympanic and. petrosquamous fissures,
2. spine of the sphenoid,
3. junction between osseous and cartilagenous parts of auditory tube, and
4. pharyngeal tubercle of the basi-occiput.

Anterior transverse line is drawn across the articular eminence along which lie the following:

1. foramen ovale,
2. foramen lacerum with posterior opening of pterygoid canal, and
3. the synchondrosis between the basi-occiput and basi-sphenoid.

30
Norma Lateralis

While examining the skull from the other aspects, some features of the side of the skull with the mandible in position have been described. Central region of norma lateralis deserves special consideration, since it is not discussed so far. This region comprises temporal fossa, zygomatic arch, external acoustic meatus, stylomastoid region, infratemporal and pterygopalatine fossae. To examine the infratemporal and pterygopalatine fossae, it may be necessary to remove the mandible and dismember the zygomatic arch.

TEMPORAL FOSSA

It lies above the zygomatic arch. The fossa is bounded above and behind by the superior temporal line, in front by the temporal surface of the zygomatic and the adjoining greater wing of sphenoid bones, below and behind by the supra-mastoid crest of temporal bone; below and in front it communicates with the infratemporal fossa through a gap between the zygomatic arch and the side of the skull.

ZYGOMATIC ARCH

It forms a palpable bony landmark, placed horizontally between the temple and the cheek. The arch is formed by:

1. temporal process of zygomatic
2. zygomatic process of temporal bones
3. zygomatic process of maxilla anteriorly. The gap between the zygomatic arch and the side of the skull transmits essentially the tendon of temporalis on its way of insertion into the coronoid process of the mandible.

Note: The inner aspects of the four angles of each parietal bone are vascular so that trephining of skull at any angle produces obvious haemorrhage. The bregma and lambda are related with superior sagittal sinus, asterion with sigmoid sinus, and pterion with anterior division of middle meningeal vessels.

The floor of the fossa is contributed by portions of:

1. the parietal,
2. greater wing of the sphenoid,
3. squamous parts of the frontal, and
4. temporal bones.

Anterior part of the floor presents a figure of H-suture known as pterion, where four bones (parietal, frontal, temporal and greater wing of sphenoid) meet; the horizontal limb of the suture is formed by the antero-inferior angle of parietal and the tip of the greater wing of sphenoid. The centre of the pterion, which is an important landmark for surgeons, lies about 4 cm above the zygomatic arch and 3.5 cm behind the fronto-zygomatic suture. Beneath the pterion lies anterior branch of middle meningeal vessels and the stem of the lateral sulcus of brain (sylvian point).

The **temporal line,** which forms the upper limit of temporal fossa, arches upward and backward from the zygomatic process of frontal bone across the parietal bone where it splits into **superior** and **inferior temporal lines.** Traced behind, the superior line fades away, but the prominent inferior line curves downward and forward across the squamous temporal as the **supra-mastoid crest** which is continuous with the posterior root of the zygomatic process. The temporalis muscle takes origin from the most of temporal fossa extending upto the inferior temporal line; the periphery of the fossa including superior temporal line gives attachment to the temporal fascia which covers the temporalis muscle.

The upper margin of the arch is sharp, and gives attachment from outside inward to:

1. the downward extension of galea aponeurotica, and
2. temporal fascia.

Mandibular fossa (already discussed in base of skull page 146)

EXTERNAL ACOUSTIC MEATUS

The bony part of external meatus is contributed by the tympanic plate and squamous part of temporal bone. Medial end of the meatus presents a tympanic sulcus which gives attachment to the peripheral margin of the tympanic membrane; the latter intervenes between the external acoustic meatus and the tympanic cavity.

The external meatus in adult measures about 2.5 cm and consists of outer cartilagenous part forming one-third and inner bony part forming two-thirds. The tympano-mastoid fissure behind the external meatus transmits the auricular branch of vagus nerve.

The supra-meatal triangle is a depression situated immediately behind and above the meatus. It is formed by the squamous temporal, and bounded above by the supra-mastoid crest, in front by the postero-superior margin of the external meatus and behind by a vertical tangent drawn along the posterior margin of the meatal orifice. The mastoid antrum lies deep to the supra-meatal triangle at a distance of about 12 to 15 mm in adult.

The **temporal line,** which forms the upper limit of temporal fossa, arches upward and backward from the zygomatic process of frontal bone across the parietal bone. Where it splits into **superior** and **inferior temporal lines.** Traced behind, the superior line fades away, but the prominent inferior line curves downward and forward across the squamous temporal as the **supra-mastoid crest** which is continuous with the posterior root of the zygomatic process. The temporalis muscle takes origin from the most of temporal fossa extending upto the inferior temporal line; the periphery of the fossa including superior temporal line gives attachment to the temporal fascia which covers the temporalis muscle.

Stylomastoid region

MASTOID PART

The mastoid part of temporal bone lies behind the external acoustic meatus and is continuous above with the squamous temporal along a line about 1 cm. below and parallel with the supra-mastoid crest. In adult the mastoid part contains numerous intercommunicating mucous-lined air cells which communicate with the tympanic cavity through the mastoid antrum. The junction of the lambdoid, parieto-mastoid and occipito-mastoid sutures, is known as the asterion. A conical projection, the mastoid process, extends downward from the lower part of the mastoid; such process is absent at birth and develops gradually after the second year.

The external surface of the mastoid part and its process is rough and extends downwords.

(a) **Styloglossus** from the anterior surface of the tip (supplied by hypoglossal nerve);
(b) **Stylohyoid** from the posterior surface midway between the base and the tip (supplied by facial nerve);
(c) **Stylopharyngeus** from the medial surface of the base (supplied by glossopharyngeal nerve).

Laterally, the styloid process is overlapped by the parotid gland and crossed by the facial nerve while passing through the gland. **Medially,** the process is related to internal carotid artery in front, internal jugular vein behind, and last four cranial nerves (9th, 10th,11th and 12th) between them.

The **stylomastoid foramen** intervenes between the styloid and mastoid processes, and cannot be seen from the lateral surface since it is overlapped by the mastoid process. The foramen transmits the facial nerve and stylomastoid artery. Absence of mastoid process in the newborn allows the stylomastoid foramen to appear at the surface; therefore the facial nerve may be injured during a surgical incision behind the pinna of the ear.

Lateral surface of mastoid process provides the attachments of the sternocleidomastoid, splenius capitis and longissimus capitis. The mastoid foramen pierces the bone close to the occipito-mastoid suture and transmits an emissary vein from the sigmoid sinus. The inner surface of the mastoid process presents a **notch** for the origin of posterior belly of digastric muscle, and further medially a **groove** for the lodgement of occipital artery.

STYLOID PROCESS

The **styloid process** of temporal is a slender projection, about 2.5 cm long, which extends downward and forward. It lies a little in front of the mastoid process and on a deeper plane. Its base is ensheathed by the lower margin of the tympanic plate.

The styloid process gives attachment to **two** ligaments **three** muscles and presents a host of important relations; hence it may be aptly described as the **styloid apparatus**. The ligaments attached to its tip are **stylohyoid and stylomandibular**; the former is attached to the lesser cornu of the hyoid bone and suspends that bone from the skull. The muscles attached to the styloid process are :

Infra-temporal fossa

It is an irregular space behind the maxilla, and communicates above with the temporal fossa through a gap between the zygomatic arch and the side of the skull.

BOUNDARIES

Roof

Roof - medial to its communication with the temporal fossa, the roof is formed by the infra-temporal surface of greater wing of the sphenoid and the adjoining part of squamous temporal. Here greater wing is pierced by the foramen ovale and foramen spinosum.

Floor

Floor is open.

Anterior wall

Anterior wall formed by the posterior surface of the body of maxilla which presents a groove in the upper part for maxiliary nerve. Between the greater wing of the sphenoid and the maxilla the fossa communicates with the orbit through the inferior orbital fissure.

Posterior wall

Posterior wall is open.

Medial wall

Medial wall - formed by the lateral pterygoid plate; a pterygo-maxillary fissure between the lateral pterygoid plate and the maxilla communicates the infra-temporal fossa with the pterygo-palatine fossa.

Lateral wall

Lateral wall - formed by the ramus and coronoid process of mandible.

Communications

Communications - Above, with **temporal** fossa, in front, with the orbit through the inferior orbital fissure; medially, with the pterygo-palatine fossa through the **pterygo-maxillary fissure**.

CONTENTS

- Lower part of temporalis, lateral and medial pterygoid muscles;
- Mandibular nerve and its branches, maxillary and chorda tympani nerves, otic ganglion and its connections.
- Maxillary artery and its branches, pterygoid venous plexus.

Pterygo-palatine Fossa

It is a pyramidal space below the apex of the orbit; the apex or edge of the fossa is directed below. The fossa should be better named as pterygo-palatino-maxillary fossa.

BOUNDARIES

- **In front** - the upper part of the posterior surface of the body of the maxilla;
- **Behind** - the root of the pterygoid process and the adjoining anterior surface of the greater wing of the sphenoid;
- **Above** - it communicates in the lateral part with the orbit through the medial end of the inferior orbital fissure. Medial to that communication, it is bounded by the body of the sphenoid and orbital process of palatine bones.
- **Below** - the apex of the fossa is closed, where anterior and posterior walls meet.

- **Medially** - the perpendicular plate of palatine bone with its orbital and sphenoidal processes.
- **Laterally** - communicates with the infratemporal fossa through the pterygo-maxillary fissure.

SPECIAL FEATURES

The fossa presents 5 openings and 2 fissures.

Openings

- Three openings in the posterior wall, named from lateral to medial side:
  - Foramen rotundum, for the maxillary nerve;
  - Anterior opening of pterygoid canal, for pterygoid vessels and nerve and vessels of the pterygoid canal (vidian)
  - Palatino-vaginal canal for pharyngeal vessels and nerve.
- One opening in the medial wall, the sphenopalatine foramen, through which the fossa communicates with the nasal cavity, and it transmits naso-palatine vessels and nerves.
- One opening at the apex of the fossa, the greater palatine canal, for the passage of greater and lesser palatine vessels and nerves.

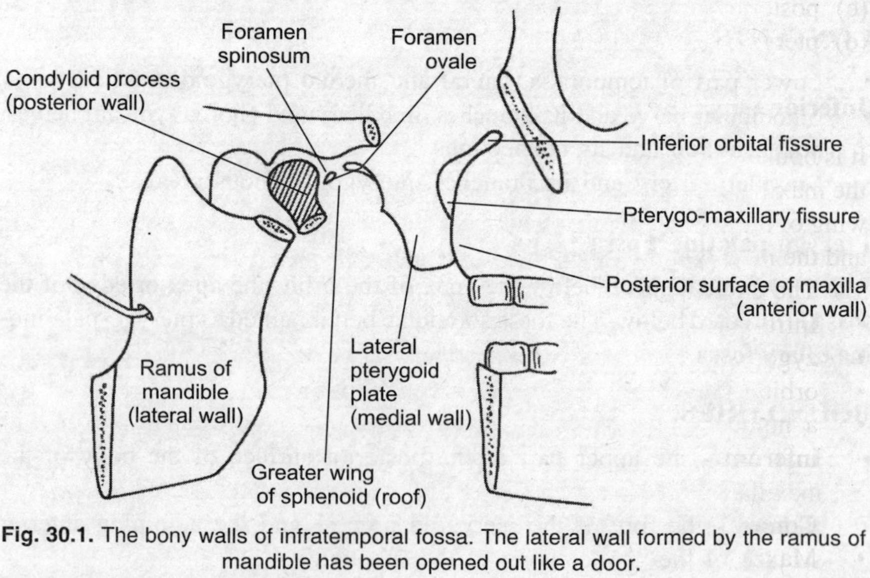

Fig. 30.1. The bony walls of infratemporal fossa. The lateral wall formed by the ramus of mandible has been opened out like a door.

FISSURE

Pterygo-maxillary Fissure

It is a triangular gap between the body of the maxilla and the anterior margin of the lateral pterygoid plate. The fissure transmits:

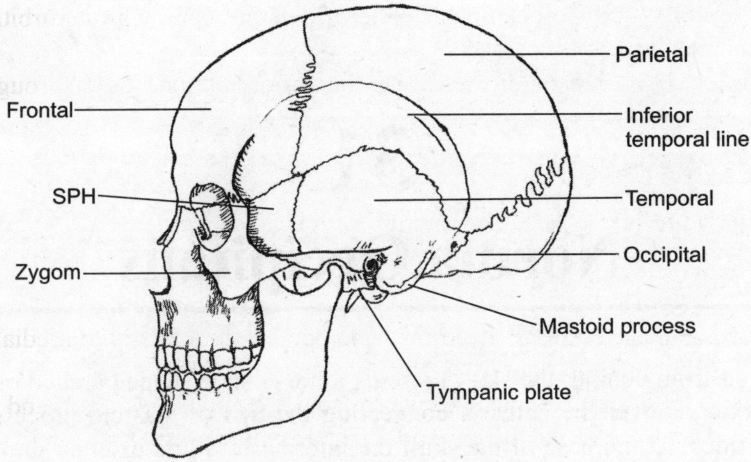

Fig. 30.2. Diagram skull in lateral view.

(a) 3rd part of maxillary artery,
(b) maxillary nerve,
(c) posterior superior alveolar vessels and nerves, and
(d) pterygoid venous plexus.

Inferior Orbital Fissure

It is bounded antero-medially by the posterior border of the orbital surface of the maxilla, postero-laterally by the lower border of orbital surface of greater wing of the sphenoid, the lateral end is limited by a notch of zygomatic bone, and the medial end by the body of the sphenoid.

The fissure transmits:

- Infra-orbital vessels and nerve;
- zygomatic branch of maxillary nerve;
- orbital branch of pterygo-palatine ganglion;
- a number of veins communicating the pterygoid venous plexus with inferior ophthalmic vein.

Contents of pterygo-palatine fossa:

- Maxillary nerve;
- Pterygo-palatine ganglion and its connections;
- Third part of maxillary artery and its branches.

31
Norma Occipitalis

Viewed from behind, the skull presents a horse-shoe shaped arched outline, and extends over the calvaria connecting the tips of mastoid processes of both sides. At the base of the skull the intermastoid line extends somewhat horizontally across the occipital condyles and foramen magnum.

The norma occipitalis is formed by parts of parietal squamous part of occipital and mastoid parts of temporal, bones. The sagittal and lambdoid sutures meet at the lambda which occupies the centre of the surface. At the lower ends of lambdoid suture, three bones (parietal, occipital and mastoid part of temporal) meet at a point which is known as the asterion. A mastoid foramen is situated close to the occipito-mastoid suture and transmits an emissary vein connecting the sigmoid sinus with the posterior auricular vein and meningeal branch of occipital artery.The external occipital protuberance is a median elevation about midway between the lambda and the foramen magnum.The most salient point of the protuberance is known as the inion. The superior nuchal lines arch bilaterally from the protuberance to the rough outer surface of the mastoid processes.These lines form the boundary between the scalp and the neck. The superior nuchal line gives attachment entirely to the investing layer of deep cervical fascia. Its medial part provides origin to the trapezius, and the lateral part receives insertion to the posterior fibres of the sternocleidomastoid and beneath that to the splenius capitis. The highest nuchal lines, when present, extend from the external protuberance above the superior nuchal lines. The highest line gives attachment medially to the galea aponeurotica, and laterally to the occipital belly of the occipitofrontalis.

The external occipital crest extends downward as a median ridge from the inion to the foramen magnum. It gives attachment to the ligamentum nuchae. From the midpoint of the external occipital crest, the inferior nuchal line curves bilaterally.

32
Norma Verticalis

Viewed from above the skull is ovoid in outline, narrower in front than behind and the maximum breadth is at the region of the parietal eminences. The calvaria or vault of the skull is formed by 4 bones :

1. squamous part of frontal bone in front,
2. squamous part of the occipital bone behind, and
3. two parietal bones between them.

Note : 3 sutures in cranial vault:

1. **sagittal suture** between the two parietal bones,
2. **coronal sutures** between the parietal and frontal bones, and
3. **lambdoid suture** between the parietals and occipital bones.In some skulls **metopic suture** persists in full or in part between the 2 halves of the frontal bone.

The meeting point between the coronal and sagittal sutures is known as the **bregma,** where a diamond shaped unossified membrane known as the **anterior fontanelle** exists in the skull of foetus and children (upto 1 ½ to 2 years).The intersection between the sagittal and lambdoid sutures is called the **lambda,** which presents unossified membrane, the **posterior fontanelle,** in foetal and neonatal skull. The vertex is the highest point of the skull and is situated on the sagittal suture a few centimetres behind the bregma. Bones forming the calvaria are ossified in membranes. The **parietal eminence** or **tuber** represents the region of maximum convexity of each parietal bone. Two ossific centres appear simultaneously in each parietal eminence in the 7th week of intrauterine life and later fuse to form a single centre, from which ossification spreads like the spokes of a wheel so that the borders of the parietal bone are ossified earlier than the angles. This produces unossified membrana gaps or fontanelles at the four angles of the parietal bones. Therefore six fontanelle are seen in both parietal bones in neonatal skull—unpaired anterior and posterior fontanelle and paired antero-lateral (sphenoidal) and postero-lateral (mastoid) fontanelle. Within 4 months after birth all fontanelles are closed by bones, except the anterior one which persists upto 18 months to 2 years after birth.

SCALP

The soft tissue including the overlying skin which covers the calvaria is called the scalp

The **cephalic index** is calculated as follows: Maximum breadth/Maximum Length × 100. When the maximum width of skull is less than 75% of its maximum length, it is called the **dolichocephalic** or long headed; more than 80% it is called the **brachycephalic** or broad headed; between 75 and 80% it is called the **mesaticephalic**.

33
The Ethmoid Bone

Median, unpaired, fragile, pneumatic (air-filled) and irregular bone, consists of horizontal cribriform plate and a lateral pair of labyrinths, each extending downward into a cuboidal, air-filled and fragile bony mass.

CRIBRIFORM PLATE

Fills up the ethmoidal notch between the two orbital plates of frontal bone. Presents a series of apertures on each side for the passage of olfactory nerves their arachnoid coverings.The plate possesses a posterior margin, and upper and lower surface; the upper surface forms the floor of the anterior cranial fossa and the lower surface the root of the nasal cavity.

The posterior margin articulates with the ethmoidal spine of the body of the sphenoid.

The upper surface presents in the median plane a triangular raised crest, the crista galli. Posterior border of crista galli is long and gives attachment to the anterior end of the falx cerebri; short anterior border of the crista diverges into two alae to join with the frontal bone and forms the posterior boundary of the foramen caecum.The perforated plate on each side of the crista galli supports the gyrus rectus of the frontal lobe and the olfactory bulb. Anterior

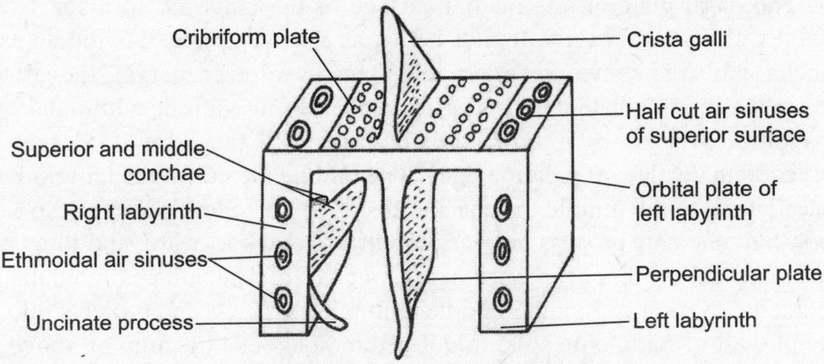

Fig. 33.1. Plan of ethmoid bone as seen from front.

part of upper surface on each side of crista presents a slit occupied by dura mater, and further laterally a small foramen for the passage of the anterior ethmoidal nerve and vessels.

The lower surface presents in the median plane a quadrilateral, perpendicular plate which projects downwards to form the upper part of the nasal septum. Anterior border of perpendicular plate slopes downward and forward, and articulates with the nasal spine of the frontal bone and with the crest formed by the union of the two nasal bones; posterior border articulates in the upper part with the sphenoidal crest and in the lower part with the vomer; inferior border is grooved to receive the septal cartilage of nose.

LABYRINTHS

Each labyrinth is cuboidal in form and contains a number of ethmoidal air-cells between the orbital plate laterally and the nasal plate medially. The ethmoidal sinuses are arranged in anterior, middle and posterior groups; in disarticulated skull the walls of some air sinuses are kept open and only to be closed when adjacent bones are assembled for articulation. The sinuses, however, communicate in the recent state with the meatuses of nasal cavity.

The upper surface of each labyrinth articulates with the broad medial margin of the orbital plate of frontal bone; anterior and posterior ethmoidal canals extend transversely across the area of articulation and transmit respectively anterior and posterior ethmoidal vessels and nerves. The anterior surface articulates with the lacrimal bone and frontal process of the maxilla, and completes the anterior ethmoidal sinuses. The posterior surface joins with the upper vertical part of sphenoidal concha and orbital process of palatine bone. The lower surface as represented by the lower margin of the orbital plate articulates with the medial margin of orbital surface of the body of maxilla.

The orbital plate is an oblong thin vertical plate which forms the medial wall of orbit, and overlaps the posterior and middle ethmoidal air-cells.

The nasal plate on the medial surface of the labyrinth forms a part of lateral wall of nasal cavity. It ends below as a curved plate, the middle nasal concha, which is convex medially and presents a lower margin; the latter is free in the intermediate part, but articulates in front with the ethmoidal crest of frontal process of maxilla and behind with the ethmoidal crest of perpendiculate plate of palatine bone. The middle meatus of the labyrinth is a space lateral to the middle concha and displays the following features : (a) A hook-like uncinate process projects downward and backward, and joins with the ethmoidal process of inferior nasal concha; (b) The bulla ethmoidalis is a rounded elevation containing middle ethmoidal air cells and projects into the lateral wall of middle meatus; middle ethmoidal cells open on or above the bulla; (c) The hiatus semilunaris is an interval between the uncinate process below and in front, and bulla ethmoidal is above and behind. A bony passage, the infundibulum, extends upward and forward within the labyrinth from the anterior part of hiatus semilunaris, receives the opening of anterior ethmoidal air cells and its tip usually communicates with the frontal sinus through the fronto-nasal duct.

Posterior part of the nasal surface above the middle nasal concha presents a narrow oblique groove, the superior meatus, which is limited above by a curved plate known as the superior nasal concha; the superior meatus receives the openings of posterior ethmoidal sinuses. The area above the superior concha and intervening between the ethmoid and the body of sphenoid is known as the spheno-ethmoidal recess, into which the sphenoidal sinus opens.

OSSIFICATION

The ethmoid bone is ossified from three centres in cartilagenous nasal capsule. one for each labyrinth, and one for the perpendicular plate.

The centres for the labyrinths appear during the fourth and fifth foetal months, and that for the perpendicular plate appear during the first year. The fusion of the three components takes place in the second year. The ethmoidal air cells develop as narrow pouches in intra-uterine life.

APPLIED ANATOMY

1. Fracture of the cribriform plate may produce rhinorrhea with the discharge of cerebrospinal fluid through the nose.
2. Fracture of ethmoidal labyrinth by crushing injuries produces a breach of separation between the orbital and nasal cavities so that the blowing the nose may produce exophthalmus. This may be associated with the spread of air bubbles in the subcutaneous tissue of eyelids and face, producing surgical emphysema.

34
The Mandible

The mandible forms the lower jaw and is the only movable bone of skull, articulating with the temporal bones at the synovial temporo-mandibular joints. It is the largest and strongest bone of the face, and consists of a horizontal horse-shoe shaped body and two broad and oblong rami projecting upward. Viewed from the side, each half of the bone is L-shaped. In the newborn, the body is composed of two halves, united at the symphysis menti by a fibrous joint which is replaced by bone within two years.

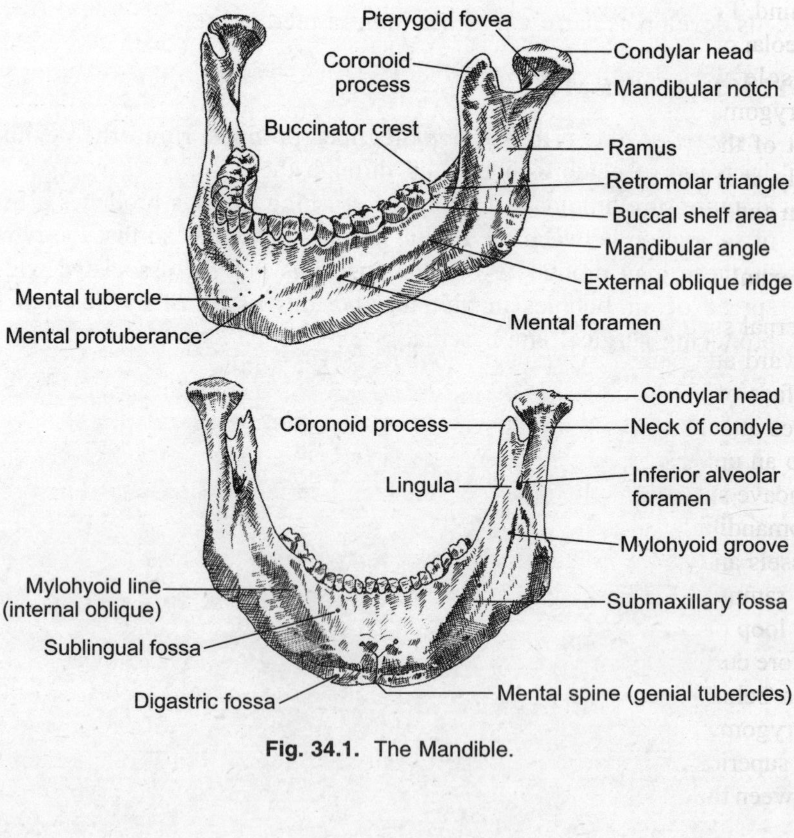

Fig. 34.1. The Mandible.

BODY

It presents external and internal surfaces, upper or alveolar border and lower border or base.

External surface

It presents at the symphysis menti a triangular mental protuberance, which is sometimes centrally depressed and exhibits mental tubercles on each side of its base. Below the incisor teeth and on each side of the protuberance lies the incisive fossa for the attachment of mentalis and a slip of orbicularis oris near the alveolar margin. The mental foramen is seen on the external surface, midway between the alveolar and lower borders (in adults) in the interval between the premolar teeth. The foramen is directed backward and laterally, and transmits mental vessels and nerve.

An oblique line extends diagonally backward and upward across this surface and below the mental foramen from the mental tubercle to the anterior border of the ramus of mandible. Anterior part of the oblique line gives attachment to depressor labii inferioris in front and to depressor anguli oris behind. Posterior part of the oblique line encroaches on the outer surface of alveolar process and opposite the 3 molar teeth provides origin to the buccinator muscle which extends behind the third molar tooth and meets the pterygomandibular raphe. The area below the oblique line is overlapped by a part of the platysma, and at the junction of the mandibular ramus and the body, it is crossed upward and forward by the tortuous facial artery, facial vein and marginal mandibular branch of facial nerve (from within outwards).

Internal surface

Internal surface on each side, an oblique mylohyoid line extends diagonally upward and backward from the lower part of symphysis menti to the inner surface of the alveolar border, a little below the third molar tooth. This line gives attachment to the mylohyoid muscle, and divides the internal surface into an upper, smooth sublingual fossa for the sublingual gland and a lower concave submandibular fossa for the lateral surface of superficial part of the submandibular gland. The mylohyoid groove conveying the corresponding vessels and nerve extends downward and forward from the inner surface of the ramus of mandible to the posterior part of submandibular fossa. Usually the loop of facial artery lodges in this *fossa* between the bone and the gland, before curling upward around the lower border of the body of mandible. The area behind the 3rd molar tooth gives attachment to the lower end of the pterygomandibular raphe, and close to the posterior end of mylohyoid line, the superior constrictor muscle. In fact the pterygomandibular raphe intervenes between the attachments of buccinator in front and superior constrictor muscle behind.The lingual nerve before reaching the tongue, comes in close contact with the inner surface of alveolar border beneath the mucoperiosteum of the gum, and intervenes between the third molar and the posterior end of mylohyoid line.

Posterior surface of symphysis menti, above the anterior ends of mylohyoid line, presents elevated pairs of superior and Inferior genial tubercles (mental spines). The superior tubercle gives attachment to the genioglossus and the inferior tubercle to the geniohyoid muscles.

Upper or alveolar border

It bears the sockets for the roots of the teeth of lower jaw. (For dental formula see the Maxillae.)

Lower border or base

It extends backwards and laterally from the symphysis menti and is continuous with the lower border of mandibular ramus behind the last molar tooth. On each side of the symphasis menti the border presents a depressed area, the digastric fossa, for the origin of anterior belly of digastric muscle. The border presents a slight sinuous curve with convexity in front and concavity behind.

The investing layer of deep cervical fascia splits into superficial and deep layers to enclose the submandibular gland. The superficial layer is attached to the entire lower border of the mandible, and the deep layer gains attachment to the mylohyoid line. The platysma muscle is attached to the lower border superficial to the investing deep fascia.

Ramus of the mandible

Each ramus is an oblong, flattened plate and extends almost vertically upward from the posterior part of the body. The ramus presents two surfaces, four borders and two processes.

Surfaces

The lateral surface is flat and monopolised for the attachment of the masseter, except the postero-superior part which is overlapped by the parotid gland. Postero-inferior part of the surface is marked by faint oblique ridges for the intramuscular septa of the masseter.

The medial surface presents close to its centre a mandibular foramen which transmits inferior alveolar vessels and nerve. The foramen leads downward and forward within the body of mandible into a mandibular canal *(see* later). Antero-medial margin of the mandibular foramen is guarded by an upward tongue-like projection, the lingula, which gives attachment to the lower end of the sphenomandibular ligament. Behind the lingula a mylohyoid groove extends downward and forward for a variable distance below the mylohyoid line and conveys mylohyoid vessels and nerve. Postero-inferior to the mylohyoid groove the medial surface extending upto the angle of mandible affords attachment to the medial pterygoid muscle; the area is sometimes marked by oblique ridges for the intermuscular septa. Above and behind the mandibular foramen, the medial surface is related to the maxillary artery (1st part) and its inferior, alveolar branch.

BORDERS AND PROCESS

The upper border displays a condylar process behind and a coronoid process in front, separated by a mandibular notch, through which masseteric vessels and nerve pass.

The condylar process carries above an expanded articular head which is convex on all sides, but transversely elliptical so that the axis of the head is set at right angles to the ramus of mandible. The head is covered by a fibro-cartilage, articulates with the anterior part of mandibular fossa of temporal bone separated by an articular disc and forms the synovial temporo-mandibular joints. A constricted neck connects the head with the ramus and bears on its antero-medial surface a depression for the insertion of the lateral pterygoid muscle. The capsular ligament of temporo-mandibular joint is attached around the neck; the lateral surface and posterior border of the neck gives attachment to the temporo-mandibular ligament. Medial surface of the neck below the attachment of capsular ligament is related to the auriculo-temporal nerve.

The coronoid process is a triangular upward projection and receives the attachment of temporalis muscle which involves the entire medial surface including its tip and anterior border and encroaching partially on its lateral surface. The coronoid process is produced by the upward pull of temporalis muscle.

The junction between the lower and posterior borders forms the angle of mandible, which measures about 110° – 115° in adults, after the eruption of permanent teeth. In edentulous newborn and in old age, after the loss of teeth, the angle is increased to about 140°. Just above the angle is attached the stylomandibular ligament, a derivative of investing layer of the deep cervical fascia. The posterior border is thick and rounded, and is overlapped by the parotid gland, which curls around the border and covers the adjoining postero-superior part of the medial and lateral surface of the ramus. The anterior border is continuous with the coronoid process and gives attachment to the temporalis muscle.

MANDIBULAR CANAL

It curves downward and forward from the mandibular foramen within the mandibular ramus and conveys the inferior alveolar vessels and nerve.

Thereafter the canal runs forward within the body below the alveolar sockets and provides branches to the roots of the teeth of lower jaw. At the interval between the first and second premolar teeth, the canal divides into mental and incisive canals. The mental canal curls upward, backward and laterally and transmits mental vessels and nerve through the mental foramen. The incisive canal conveying the corresponding vessels and nerve extends further forward to supply the canine and incisor teeth.

Ossification

The mandible is the second bone in the body to start ossification after the clavicle. Each half of the bone is ossified in the 6th week of intra-uterine life mostly in membrane forming the fibrous envelope of the Meckel's cartilage (of first branchial arch) the cartilage cells being absorbed. The membranous ossification involves roughly the area extending from the mandibular to the mental foramina. In front of the mental foramen the ossification takes place directly from the same centre in the ventral end of the Meckel's cartilage and is represented by the mental ossicles.The ramus above the mandibular foramen is ossified from secondary cartilages, attached to the Meckel's cartilage as an extension from the same ossific centre; these parts include the condylar and coronoid processes.

The two halves of the mandibular body are united by a fibrous joint at the symphysis menti, which is replaced by bone within the second year.

At birth

At birth, the body of edentulous mandible is full of teeth and consequently the mental foramen and mandibular canal lie close to its lower border. Eruption of deciduous or milk teeth commences usually in the 6th post-natal month and is complete during the second year. In the newborn, the angle of mandible is obtuse (140°) and the coronoid process lies at a higher level than the condylar process.

In Adults

In adults, after eruption of the permanent teeth the mental foramen lies midway between the upper and lower borders of the bone. Growth of the rami takes place both posteriorly and vertically by a process of remodelling. Posterior growth accommodates the eruption of permanent molar teeth and reduces the angle of mandible to about 110° - 115°. Vertical growth allows the condylar process to be higher than the coronoid process. In old age, after the loss of teeth, absorption of the alveolar margin brings the mental foramen nearer the upper border of the mandible and exposes the mental nerve to the pressure of artificial denture.

After complete absorption of the alveolar wall, a linear alveolar ridge is laid down in both maxillae and mandible. In the maxillae, the labial wall of all alveolar sockets is thinner and after absorption, the alveolar ridge lies entirely within the line of teeth in the mandible, the labial wall of the alveolar sockets for the incisor and canine teeth is thinner, whereas in the molar sockets the lingual wall is thinner. Therefore, after absorption of the sockets the curve of the alveolar ridge is narrower in front and lies within the line of front teeth, and wider behind lying outside the line of molar teeth.This knowledge is important for dental surgeons during the setting of artificial dentures.

Some important observations on the mandible:

- **Attachments of ligaments**: Capsule of temporo-mandibular joint around the neck; temporo-mandibular ligament on the lateral and posterior surfaces of the neck; sphenomandibular ligament at the lingula; pterygomandibular raphe behind the third molar tooth; stylomandibular ligament just above the angle of mandible.
- **Relations of nerves:** Lingual nerve on the medial side of the alveolar border slightly below the third molar and above the posterior end of mylohyoid line; inferior alveolar nerve in the mandibular foramen; mylohyoid nerve lodging in the corresponding groove; auriculotemporal nerve on the medial side of the neck; masseteric nerve in the mandibular notch; marginal mandibular branch of facial nerve on the outer surface of the body at the antero-inferior angle of masseter; mental nerve emerging through the corresponding foramen.
- **Relations of arteries:** Facial artery loops forward and downward between the submandibular fossa and the gland, then winds around the lower border of the mandibular body at the antero-inferior angle of the masseter and appears tortuously upward and forward in the face; first

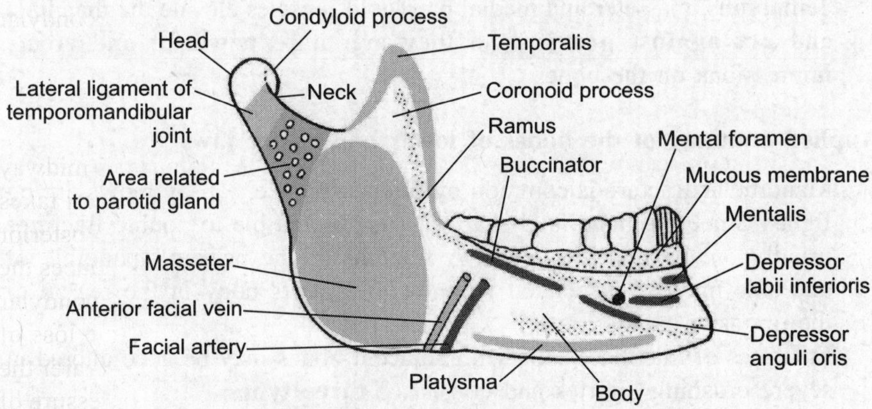

Fig. 34.2. The mandible : Lateral view of right half.

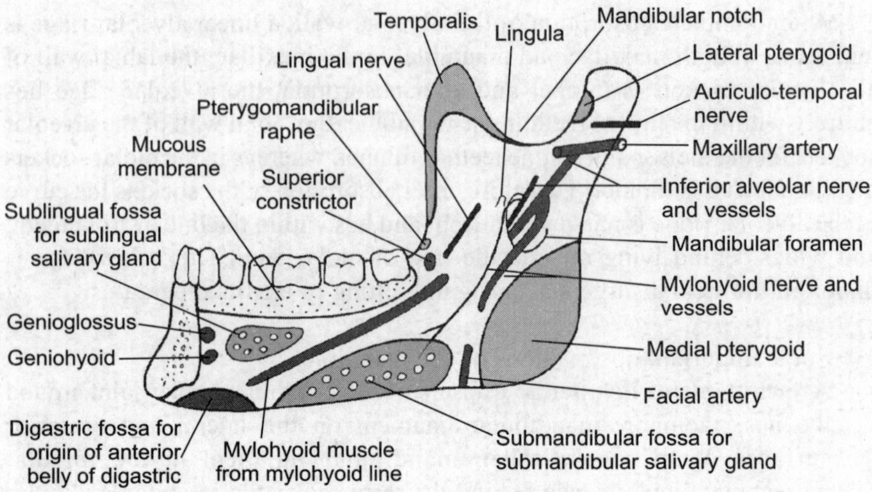

Fig. 34.3. The mandible : Medial view of right half.

part of maxillary artery on the medial side of the neck; other arteries accompany the corresponding nerves.

- **Relations of salivary glands:** Parotid gland curls around the posterior border and overlaps the adjoining postero-superior part of lateral and medial surfaces of ramus of mandible; superficial part of submandibular gland in the submandibular fossa; sublingual gland in the sublingual fossa.
- **Attachments of muscles of masticatlon: Temporalis** on the entire coronoid process; **masseter** on the outer surface of the ramus; **medial pterygoid** on the inner surface of the ramus; **lateral pterygoid** in front of the neck of mandible.

  Temporalis, masseter and medial pterygoid muscles elevate the mandible and **act against gravity.** So they are more powerful and create impressions on the bone.

Applied anatomy of the bones of lower and upper jaws

- Mandibular fracture is common by direct violence, *e.g.* by blows during fights. Since the bone is U-shaped, it is susceptible to double fractures usually on the opposite sides. A fracture of the neck of mandible of one side may be associated with fracture of its body in the region of the opposite canine tooth.
- Fractures of maxillae along with adjacent bones may be encountered in severe crushing injuries and consist of **three types**:
  - **Le Fort I -** Both maxillae may be fractured transversely at the level of nasal floor, and the upper jaw becomes movable.

- **Le Fort II -** The fractures involve the postero-Iateral parts of maxillary sinuses and extend across the infra-orbital part of the bridge of nose. In such condition the entire central part of the face is separated from the rest of the skull. This is associated with **CSF rhinorrhoea** due to fracture of ethmoid bone and tearing of the meninges.
- **Le Fort III -** This is a severe form of horizontal fracture that separates the splanchnocranium from the neurocranium and allows the face to move posteriorly and obstruct the airway.

35
The Nasal Bones

A pair of small, stout nasal bones and form the upper part of the bridge of nose. Each bone is triagular in outline, with the truncated apex directed above.

It presents:

1. an apex, 2. a base,

2 borders:

1. lateral, 2. medial

2 surfaces:

1. outer, 2. inner.

The apex is thick, serrated and articulates with the nasal notch of frontal bone.

The base is thin, notched and continuous with the lateral nasal cartilage. The foramen between them transmits the external nasal nerves as a continuation of anterior ethmoidal nerve.

The lateral border joins with the frontal process of the maxilla.

The medial border is thick above and thin below, articulates with its fellow and forms internally a nasal crest; the latter articulates from above downwards with the nasal spine of frontal and perpendicular plate of ethmoid bones.

The outer surface is convex from side to side and concave from above downward, and presents near its centre a foramen through which a vein passes from the nasal mucous membrane. The surface is covered by the procerus and a part of nasalis muscles.

The inner (nasal) surface is concave, covered by the mucous membrane and is traversed by a longitudinal groove for the anterior ethmoidal nerve.

OSSIFICATION

The nasal bone is ossified in membrane from a single centre which appears in the 3rd Intra-uterine month.

APPLIED ANATOMY

Fracture of the nasal bones is fairly common by a blow on the nose. This is associated with nasal bleeding.

36
The Occipital Bone

It is a curved plate of bone, concave internally, somewhat trapezoid in outline, and occupies the posterior part of the vault and the base of cranial cavity . The bone presents in the median plane the foramen magnum, which divides the bone into four parts: an expanded plate of squamous part curving backward and upward, a basilar part projecting forward and upward, and a pair of condylar parts lateral to the foramen.

Anatomical position: Keeping the foramen magnum in horizontal plane, the basilar part is directed forward and upward.

Squamous part (squama): It presents external and internal surfaces, a pair of supero-lateral or lambdoid borders, a pair of infero-lateral or mastoid borders, and three angles-superior and two lateral. External surface it is convex and presents a median elevation, the external occipital protuberance, about

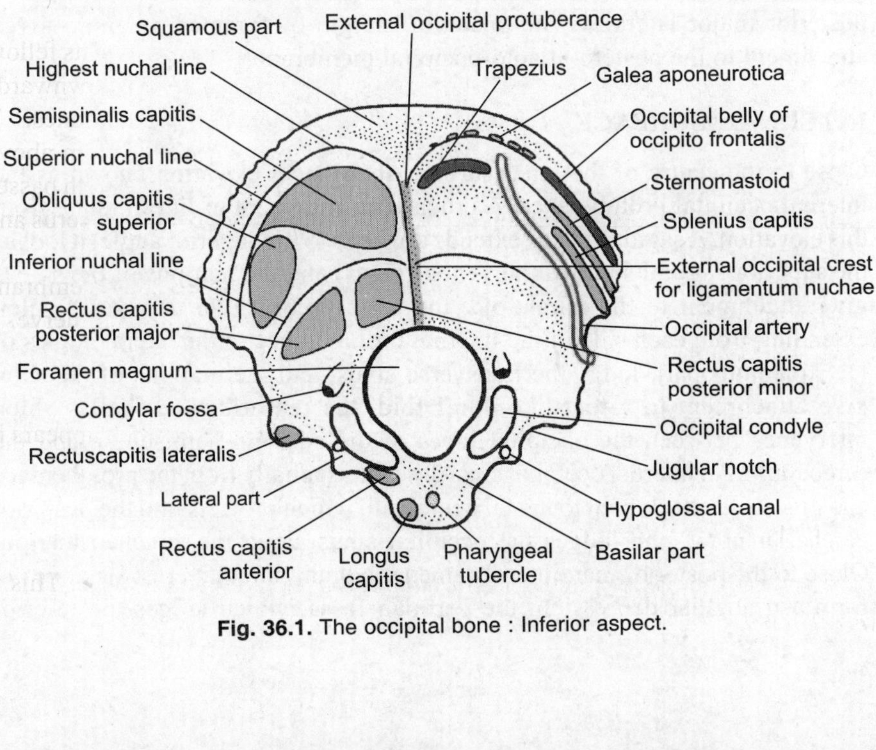

Fig. 36.1. The occipital bone : Inferior aspect.

midway between the superior angle and the foramen magnum. The most prominent point of the protuberance is known as the inion. The superior nuchal lines arch bilaterally with upward convexity from the protuberance to the outer surface of the mastoid part of temporal bones. The investing layer of deep cervical fascia is attached to the entire extent of superior nuchal line; the medial part of the line provides origin to the trapezius, and the lateral part receives insertions of the posterior fibres of sternocleidomastoid and beneath it to the splenius capitis. The superior nuchal lines form the boundary between the scalp and the neck and divides the squamous part of the bone into an upper planum occipitale and a lower planum nuchale. A pair of highest nuchal lines arch laterally above the superior lines from the external protuberance. The highest lines give attachment medially to the galea aponeurotica and laterally to the occipital belly of occipitofrontalis. The area of the bone above the highest lines is smooth and covered by occipito-frontalis on each side and galea aponeurotica (epicranial aponeurosis) between them.

A median ridge known as the external occipital protuberance extends downwards from the inion to the foramen magnum. It gives upper attachment to the ligament nuchae.

The inferior nuchal lines curve bilaterally from the midpoint of the external occipital crest. The area between the superior and the inferior nuchael lines provides insertion on each side of the crest to the semispinalis capitis medially and to the obliquus capitis superior laterally. The area between the inferior nuchal lines and the posterior margin of foramen magnum receives on each side insertion of the rectus capitis posterior minor medially and rectus capitis posterior major laterally. The posterior margin of foramen magnum gives attachment to the postero-atlanto-occipital membrane.

INTERNAL SURFACE

Close to the centre of the inner surface, there is an elevation known as the internal occipital protuberance. A cruciate arrangement of lines radiate from this elevation. A sagittal sulcus extends upwards to the superior angle; it lodges the superior sagittal sinus (dural venous sinus) and the margins of the sulcus give attachment to the dural fold, the falx cerebri. Two transverse sulci, extending from each side of the internal protuberance to the lateral angles of the squamous part, lodge the transverse sinus, and the margins of the sulci give attachment to a tent-like dural fold, the tentorium cerebelli, which intervenes between the occipital lobes of the cerebral hemisphere and the cerebellum. An internal occipital crest descends sagitally from the protuberance and gives rise attachment to the falx cerebelli, which projects into the posterior cerebeller notch and lodges the occipital sinus along the attached margin. Close to the posterior margin of foramen magnum, internal crest separates to form a triangular depression, the vermian fossa, which lodges the inferior vermis of cerebellum. The confluence of venous sinuses (torcula Hirophili) is located at the internal occipital protuberance, where superior sagittal sinus is usually continuous with the right transverse sinus, and the straight sinus with left transverse sinus. Le Gross Clerk suggested that in right-handed individual the superior sagittal sinus is continuous with the right transverse sinus, in left-handed person with the left transverse sinus and in amphidextrous individual with both transverse sinuses. However, this statement does not receive much acceptance due to lack of evidence.

The squamous part is divided by the cruciate lines into four fossae : upper two triangular fossae for the occipital lobes of cerebral hemispheres. and lower two quadrilateral fossae for accommodation of the cerebellar hemispheres.

Supero-lateral borders (lambdoid)

Each border is serrated and articulates with the posterior border of parietal bone, and forms half of the lambdoid suture.

Infero-lateral borders (mastoid)

Each border extends from the lateral angle to the jugular process and is serrated for articulation with the posterior border of mastoid part of the corresponding temporal bone.

Superior angle

It is meeting point of the sagittal and lambdoid sutures and is known as lambda,

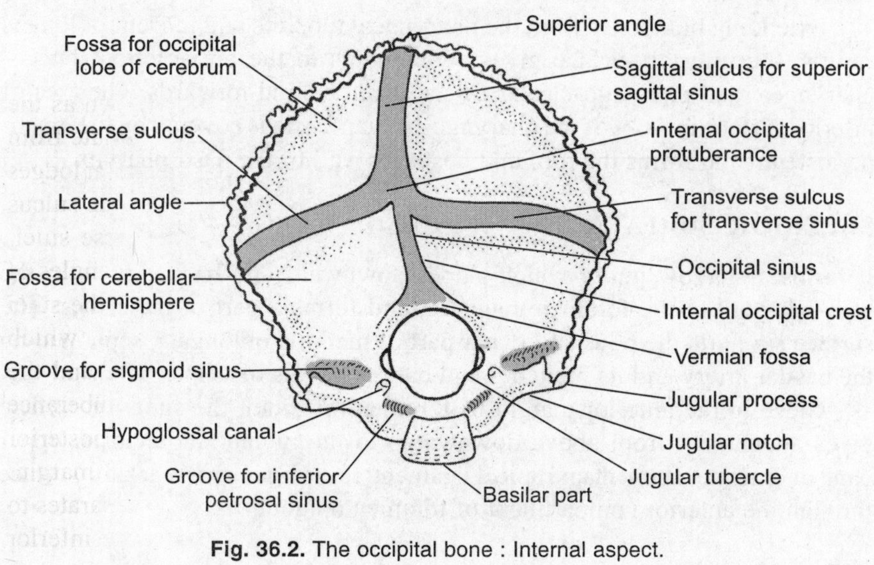

Fig. 36.2. The occipital bone : Internal aspect.

where the occipital bone meets with both parietal bones. The posterior fontanelle is located here in foetal skull.

Lateral angles

Each angle is the meeting place between occipital, parietal and mastoid part of temporal bones, and is known as the asterion, where a postero-lateral fontanelle is present in foetal skull.

BASILAR PART (BASI-OCCIPUT)

It extends forward and upward from the anterior margin of foramen magnum upto the body of sphenoid bone. The basilar part presents three surfaces—anterior, inferior and superior, and two lateral borders.

Anterior surface: It is quadrilateral, rough and articulates by a plate of hyaline cartilage with the posterior surface of body of sphenoid bone, forming a primary cartilagenous joint (synchondrosis) which is replaced by bone (synostosis) usually after 25 years.

Inferior surface: It faces downward and forward, and presents a pharyngeal tubercle in the median plane about 1 cm in front of foramen magnum. The pharyngeal tubercle gives attachment to the upper end of fibrous raphe of the pharynx, where the constrictor muscles of pharynx are inserted. A depression on each side of the tubercle receives the insertion of longus capitis. Close to the anterior end of occipital condyles, the inferior surface provides insertion to the rectus capitis anterior in a depressed area.

The anterior margin of foramen magnum gives attachment to the anterior atlanto-occipital membrane.

Extending bilaterally from the pharyngeal tubercle and in front of longus capitis, the inferior surface gives attachments to the prevertebral, bucco-pharyngeal and pharyngo-basilar fasciae from behind forwards. The area of inferior surface in front of the pharyngo-basilar fascia is covered by the muco-periosteum and forms the roof and posterior wall of the naso-pharynx.

SUPERIOR SURFACE

It forms a shallow gutter which slopes downward and backward from the basi-sphenoid to the foramen magnum, and forms a part of the clivus. The surface supports the pons and upper part of medulla oblongata, separated by the basilar artery and its branches and basilar plexus of veins.

Close to the anterior margin of foramen magnum, the superior surface gives attachment from above downwards to the membrana tectoria, upper band of cruciate ligament and apical ligament; these ligaments reach the surface through the anterior compartment of foramen magnum.

LATERAL BORDERS

Each border articulates with the medial part of posterior border of petrous part of temporal bone by sutural ligaments. A groove along the upper surface of the line of articulation lodges the inferior petrosal sinus, which is the first tributary of internal jugular vein.

CONDYLAR PARTS

Each is situated by the side of foramen magnum, and consists of condylar part proper and jugular process.

Condylar part (Proper) - Inferior surface presents an obliquely placed, convex articular surface, the occipital condyle, which occupies the anterior half of the outer margin of foramen magnum. The condyle converges in front to the undersurface of the basi-occiput; the articular surface is oval or reniform in outline, faces downward and laterally, and articulates with the superior articular facet of the lateral mass of atlas forming the synovial atlanto-occipital joint. The medial margin of the occipital condyle presents a tubercle which projects into the side of foramen magnum for the attachment of alar ligaments. The hypoglossal canal lies above the articular condyle at its junction of anterior one-third and posterior two-thirds, and extends antero-laterally from an inner opening a little above the lateral margin of foramen magnum. The canal transmits the hypoglossal nerve, meningeal branch of ascending pharyngeal artery and sometimes emissary veins; occasionally the canal is divided by a spicule of bone into two or more compartments. Just behind the condyle lies a depression, the condylar fossa, for accommodation of the up-turned posterior margin of the superior articular facet of the atlas, during full extension of the head at the atlanto-occipital joint. Sometimes a posterior condylar canal affects the floor of the condylar fossa on one or both sides; the canal transmits an emissary vein connecting the sigmoid sinus with the sub-occipital venous plexus.

Superior surface of the condylar part presents a jugular tubercle (tuberculum jugulare) which bridges over the hypoglossal canal. Posterior part of the tubercle is marked by faint oblique grooves for the passage of glossopharyngeal, vagus and accessory nerves through the intermediate compartment of jugular foramen.

JUGULAR PROCESS

Each process projects laterally as a quadrilateral plate from the posterior half of occipital condyle, and presents anterior and lateral margins, lower and upper surfaces.

The anterior margin presents a concave, free jugular notch which forms posterior boundary of jugular foramen and transmits internal jugular vein as a continuation of sigmoid sinus.

The lateral margin bears a rough articular surface which joins with the corresponding jugular area on the undersurface of petrous-temporal bone by a plate of cartilage; the cartilagenous joint is replaced by bone usually after 25 years.

The lower surface of the jugular process is rough and receives insertion of the rectus capitis lateralis. Sometimes a paramastoid process extends downward from the lower surface and may articulate with the transverse process of atlas.

The upper surface of jugular process is deeply grooved for the terminal part of sigmoid sinus, before the latter turns downward around the jugular notch and leaves through the jugular foramen as the internal jugular vein.

FORAMEN MAGNUM

It is a large oval aperture of the occipital bone and communicates the posterior cranial fossa with the vertebral canal. The middle point of anterior margin of the foramen is known as the basion.

OSSIFICATION

The occipital bone is principally ossified from eight centres: one for the basilar part, one for each condylar part, four for the squamous part, and one for the posterior margin of foramen magnum. The basilar part is ossified in cartilage in the sixth week of intra-uterine life. Each condylar part starts ossification in cartilage in the eighth prenatal week.

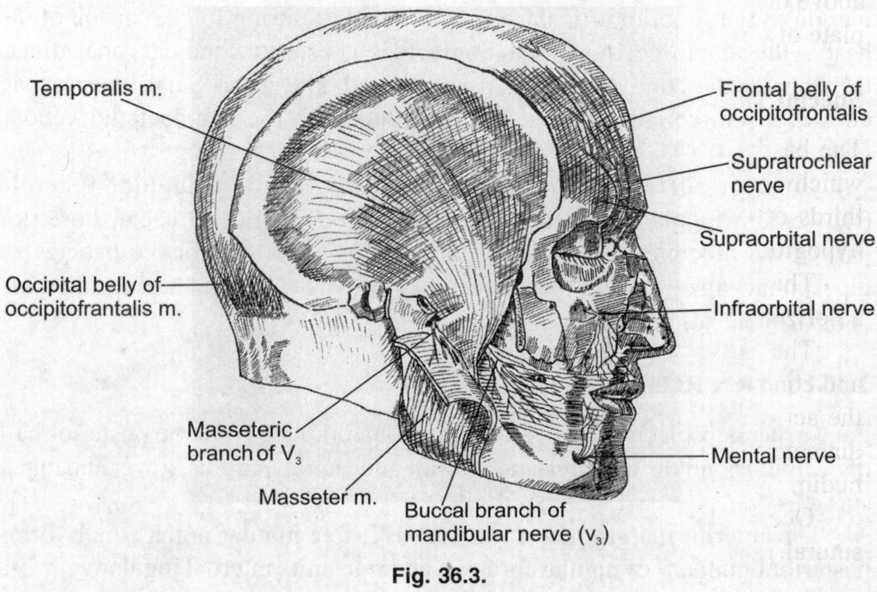

Fig. 36.3.

The squamous part below the highest nuchal line is ossified in cartilage from two centres, one on each side, in the seventh prenatal week and soon join with each other. Above the highest nuchal line, it is ossified in membrane from two bilaterally placed centres in about eighth prenatal week; these two regions of squamous part usually unite in the third month after birth.

Sometimes the part above the highest nuchal line remains separate and persists as inter-parietal bone. An occasional centre appears for the posterior margin of foramen magnum (Kerckring's centre) in the sixteenth prenatal week.

The fusion between the squamous and condylar parts takes place at about the end of second year. Within six years the basilar part fuses with the condylar parts; therefore by the sixth year the bone forms one entity. Between the eighteenth and twenty-fifth years, the occipital bone is ossiously connected with the body of sphenoid bone.

MORPHOLOGY

Morphologically, the occipital bone is formed by the fusion of three or four pre-cervical vertebrae.

The basi-occiput represents the fused body of occipital vertebrae.

The ex-occiput is formed by the jugular processes which represent the fused transverse processes of pre-cervical vertebrae, and the hypoglossal canal symbolises the intervertebral foramina.

The supra-occiput is formed by the squamous part upto the highest nuchal line, and represents the fused laminae of the pre-cervical veretebrae. The area above the highest nuchal line is a separate component derived from the tectal plate of otic capsule.

Special features of occipital bone

The basilar part is separated from the condylar parts by an imaginary line which extends across the junction of anterior one-third and posterior two-thirds of the occipital condyles; traced above, the line passes through the hypoglossal canals and bisects the jugular tubercles.

The junction between the squamous and condylar parts is represented by a horizontal line passing through the posterior ends of occipital condyles.

The primary cartilagenous joints intervening between the basi-occiput and condylar parts permit additional flexion of the foetal skull and facilitate the act of parturition through the lower part of birth-canal by reducing the diameter of foetal head; these joints are called the obstetrical hinge joints of budin.

Occipital bone presents three types of extrinsic articulations: fibrous or sutural joints at the peripheral margins, primary cartilagenous joints at the junction of the basi-occiput and basi-sphenoid, and at the junction of jugular processes and petrous temporal, and a pair synovial atlanto-occipital joints; Cartilagenous joint between the basi-occiput and the basi-sphenoid regulates the growth in length of the base of skull, and those between the jugular processes and petrous-temporal regulate the growth of the width of the skull.

Deep cervical fascia is attached to the bone in two places : investing layer along the superior nuchal lines and prevertebral layer on the inferior surface of the basi-occiput. The undersurface of the basilar part in front of pharyngeal tubercle is covered by the muco-periosteum and forms the roof and posterior wall of the nasopharynx. Venous sinuses related to the bone are: posterior part of the superior sagittal sinus a pair of transverse sinuses, occipital sinus, terminal parts of sigmoid sinuses and inferior petrosal sinus.

The nerves related to the bone are:

(a) glosso-pharyngeal (IX), vagus (X) and accessory (XI) across the jugular tubercle;
(b) hypoglossal (XII) through the hypoglossal canal;
(c) spinal root of accessory nerve through the foramen magnum;
(d) greater occipital, lesser occipital nerves on each side of external occipital protuberance.

37

The Sphenoid Bone

It is an unpaired pneumatic irregular bone, situated in the base of the skull, and wedged between the frontal and ethmoid bones in front, basi-occiput and petrous part of temporal bones behind.

It consists of a central body, and pairs of greater and lesser wings and pterygoid processes. It resembles a bat with outstretched wings and standing on pterygoid processes which represent its legs.

BODY

It is cuboidal in shape and contains a pair of sphenoidal air sinuses, separated by a median partition which is usually deflected to one side. The body presents six surfaces—superior, inferior, anterior, posterior and a pair of lateral surfaces.

1. Superior (cerebral) surface presents from before backwards the following features :
   – ***Ethmoidal spine:*** It forms a triangular projection between the two lesser wings and articulates with the posterior margin of the cribriform plate of ethmoid bone.

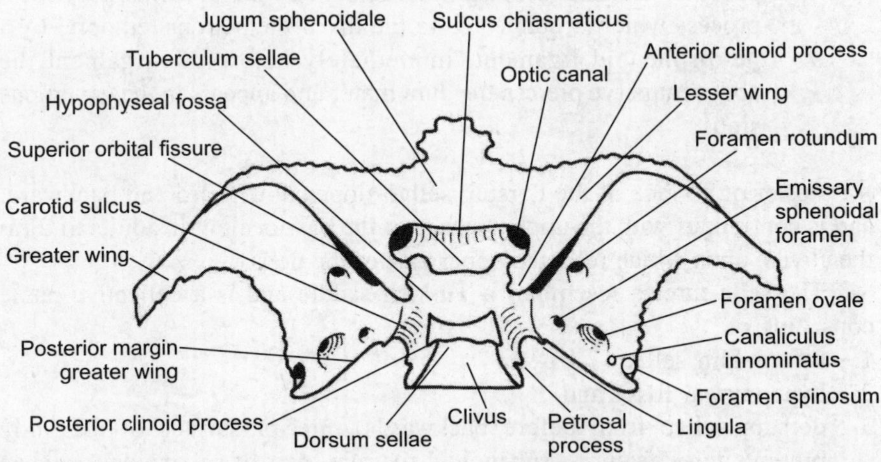

Fig. 37.1. Sphenoid bone : Superior aspect.

- ***Jugum sphenoidale:*** It is a flattened plate of bone upon which rest on each side gyrus rectus of the frontal lobe and olfactory tract.
- ***Sulcus chiasmaticus:*** It is a shallow transverse groove which leads on each side to the optic canal. Anterior part of the optic chiasma lies slightly above the sulcus.
- ***Tuberculum sellae:*** It is the posterior limit of the sulcus chiasmaticus, and gives anterior attachment to the diaphragma sellae which forms the dural roof of the hypophyseal fossa presents a small projection, the middle clinoid process, which is connected to the anterior clinoid process by the carotido-clinoid ligament. The carotido-clinold foramen thus formed between the ligament and the body of sphenoid transmits upturned internal carotid artery. A central depressed area lodges the hypophysis cerebri.
- ***Hypophyseal fossa:*** It is a deep depression which contains the hypophysis cerebri or pituitary gland. The floor of this fossa is related to the sphenoidal sinuses.

  A small median cranio-pharyngeal canal is occasionally observed in the floor of the fossa and is believed to represent a remnant of Rathke's pouch from which the anterior lobe of pituitary gland is developed.
- ***Dorsum sellae:*** It is a square-like plate of bone which projects upward and presents a conical projection, the posterior clinoid process, on each side; the latter gives attachment to the anterior end of the attached margin of tentorium cerebelli and is connected with the anterior clinoid process of the lesser wing by the interclinoid ligament. The upper margin of dorsum sellae provides posterior attachment to the diaphrgma sellae. Below the posterior clinoid process, the lateral margin of dorsum sellae presents a petrosal process which is connected to the tip of the petrous temporal by a petrosphenoid ligament; immediately below this ligament the abducent nerve pierces the dura mater and appears in the cavernous sinus.

Posterior surface of the dorsum sellae slopes downward and backward, and is continuous with the upper surface of the basi-occiput in adults to form the clivus, upon which rests the upper part of the pons.

The sella turcica resembles a Turkish saddle and is a collective name consisting of:

1. tuberculum sellae,
2. hypophyseal fossa and
3. dorsum sellae from before backwards. Inferior surface of the body presents three features: sphenoidal rostrum, pair of sphenoidal conchae (lower part) and vaginal processes.

Sphenoidal rostrum projects downward as a median ridge and is continuous with the lower end of sphenoidal crest (vide infra). It articulates with the grooved upper margin of the vomer between the diverging alae.

Lower horizontal part of each sphenoidal concha extends backward as a triangular plate by the side of the rostrum and articulates with the upper surface of the alae of vomer.

The vaginal process projects downward and medially as a narrow triangular shelf from the base of each medial pterygoid plate and lies below the horizontal part of the concha. Upper surface of the vaginal process articulates with the lateral margin of the alae of the vomer in an overlapping manner and forms a vomero-vaginal canal which does not transmit any significant structure. Anterior margin of the vaginal process and the adjoining lower surface articulate with the upper surface of sphenoidal process of palatine bone and form the palatino-vaginal (pharyngeal) canal which transmits pharyngeal vessels and nerve. Therefore, vomero-vaginal canal lies above, and palatino-vaginal canal below the vaginal process.

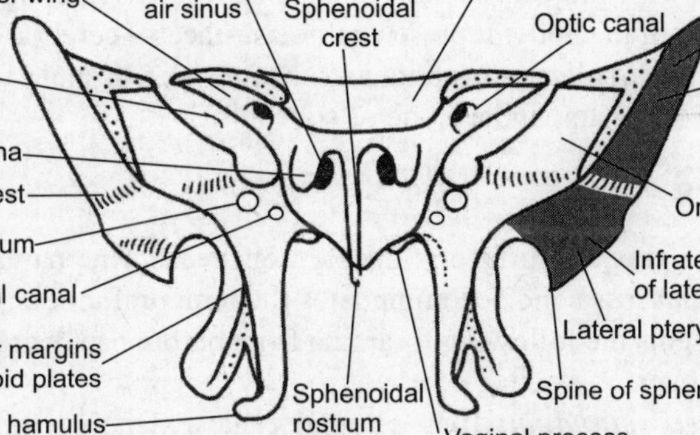

Fig. 37.2. Sphenoid bone : Anterior aspect

Anterior surface of the body presents three features : sphenoidal crest, a pair of sphenoidal conchae (upper vertical part) and articular rough area involving each concha.

Sphenoidal crest is placed vertically as a median ridge, articulates with the posterior border of perpendicular plate of ethmoid bone and forms a part of nasal septum.

Upper vertical parts of sphenoidal conchae lie on each side of the crest and complete the anterior surface of the body. Lower and medial part of each concha is smooth and presents a sphenoidal foramen, through which each sphenoidal sinus communicates with the sphenoethmoidal recess of the superior meatus of nasal cavity.

Above and lateral to the sphenoidal foramen, a quadrilateral or triangular rough area occurs on each concha, and articulates with the posterior surface of the labyrinth of ethmoid and orbital process of the palatine bones.

Posterior surface of the body is rough and quadrilateral, and articulates by a plate of hyaline cartilage with the anterior surface of the basi-occiput forming a primary cartilaginous joint which is replaced by bone usually between 20 and 25 years. If bony fusion takes place at an earlier age, say at 15 years, then the antero-posterior growth of the base of skull will be arrested so that the maxillary teeth of upper jaw fail to adjust with the teeth of lower jaw.

Above the root of greater wing, the lateral surface is marked by an italic *"f"* shaped curved groove, the carotid sulcus for the accommodation of the internal carotid artery surrounded by a plexus of sympathetic nerves. It is also related with the cavernous sinus and a series of structures within it.

The carotid sulcus is more deep in the posterior part, because it is overhung medially by the petrosal process and laterally by a raised margin. the lingula.

GREATER WINGS

Each greater wing projects laterally and then upward as a strong curved process from the side of the body. It presents three surfaces—cerebral (upper), lateral and orbital; two borders—posterior and squamosal; a tip and a triangular rough area medial to the tip, and a spine of sphenoid.

SURFACES

The cerebral (upper) surface is deeply concave, forms part of the floor of middle cranial fossa and accommodates the temporal lobe of the brain. This surface presents the following foramina from before backwards arranged in a crescentic line :

1. ***Foramen rotundum:*** It is a round canal extending forward from the middle cranial fossa to the pterygo-palatine fossa, and transmits the maxillary nerve.
2. ***Foramen ovale:*** It is a fairly large oval aperture lying posterolateral to the foramen rotundum and opens into the infra-temporal fossa. The foramen ovale transmits : sensory part of mandibular nerve along with motor root of trigeminal nerve (before forming the mandibular nerve trunk in the infra-temporal fossa), accessory meningeal artery, lesser (superficial) petrosal nerve (occasional). emissary veins connecting cavernous sinus with pterygoid venous plexus, and sometimes the anterior trunk of middle meningeal sinus.
3. ***Foramen splnosum:*** It lies close to and postero-lateral to oval foramen-separated by a bar of bone, and transmits middle meningeal artery, nervus spinosus and occasionally the posterior trunk of middle meningeal sinus.

4. ***Canaliculus Innominatus:*** It is occasionally present in the bony bar between the foramina spinosum and ovale, and transmits the lesser petrosal nerve, which then does not pass through the foramen ovale in such condition.

Emissary sphenoidal foramen (foramen Vesalii)

It is occasionally found medial to foramen ovale, and gives passage to the emissary vein connecting the cavernous sinus to the pterygoid venous plexus.

The outer surface of each greater wing is divided by a horizontal infra-temporal crest into upper and lower areas. The upper area forms a part of temporal fossa and gives origin to the temporalis muscle. The lower area including the infra-temporal crest forms the roof of the infra-temporal fossa and gives origin to the upper head of lateral pterygoid muscle.

The orbital surface of the greater wing is smooth, quadrilateral and forms the posterior part of lateral wall of the orbit. Its upper and lateral margins are articular, join respectively with the orbital plate of frontal bone and the postero-medial margin of zygomatic bone. Lower and medial margins of the orbital surface are free and non-articular. The lower margin forms the postero-lateral boundary of the inferior orbital fissure. The medial margin forms the infero-lateral boundary of the superior orbital fissure which is a retort-shaped interval between the greater and lesser wings of the sphenoid. A small tubercle of the medial margin gives attachment to a common tendinous ring, which extends across the superior orbital fissure and gains attachment around the upper and medial margins of the optic canal on the undersurface of the lesser wing.

BORDERS

The posterior border of each greater wing is non-articular in medial part and articular in the lateral part. The medial part forms the anterior boundary of foramen lacerum and presents the posterior opening of pterygoid canal transmitting pterygoid vessels and nerve. The foramen lacerum is bounded posteriorly by the apex of petrous temporal and is occupied by the anterior opening of carotid canal through which the internal carotid artery emerges and appears in the carotid sulcus after passing through the upper opening of foramen lacerum. (For further details see the norma basalis). The lateral part of the posterior border articulates with the anterior border of petrous-temporal; along the line of articulation a sulcus tubae is formed in the exterior of the base of the skull for the lodgement of the cartilagenous of the auditory tube.

The squamosal border of greater wing articulates with the antero-inferior of the squamous part of temporal bone.

The tip of greater wing is bevelled on the inner surface and overlaps the sphenoidal angle of the corresponding parietal bone forming the region of pterion. The triangular rough area medial to the tip articulates with the frontal bone.

Spine of the sphenoid

It is a small pointed process projecting downward from the junction of posterior and squamosal borders of greater wing. The spine provides the attachments to three ligaments, two muscles, and to important structures on its medial and lateral sides.

The ligaments are:

1. sphenomandibular, extending from the spine to the mandibular foramen; it is developed from the fibrous envelope of Meckel's cartilage of the first branchial arch, cartilage cells being absorbed.
2. anterior ligament of malleus, extends from the anterior process of malleus to the spine after passing through the medial end of petrotympanic fissure;
3. pterygospinous, extends from the spine to a tubercle at the posterior border of the lateral pterygoid plate.

The muscle attached to the spine are:

1. tensor veil palatini, arising from anterior margin and adjoining medial surface;
2. tensor tympani, arising from medial surface and the adjoining posterior margin. Relations of the spine: Medially, cartilagenous part of auditory tube and chorda tympani nerve; laterally, auriculo-temporal nerve.

APPLIED ANATOMY

Fracture of sphenoidal spine is manifested by secreto-motor paralysis of all (three) salivary glands on the affected side, along with loss of taste sensation from the anterior two-thirds of the corresponding half of the tongue.

Lesser wings

Each wing is a triangular plate of bone projecting laterally from the upper and anterior part of the side of the body, and connected to the latter by anterior and posterior roots which enclose between them and the sphenoidal body the optic canal. The optic canal transmits optic nerve and ophthalmic artery, inferolateral to the nerve.

The lesser wing presents anterior and posterior borders, and upper and lower surfaces.

The anterior border articulates with the posterior margin of the orbital plate of the frontal bone. The posterior border is free and concave, forms the junction of the floor between anterior and middle cranial fossae, and projects into the stem of the lateral sulcus of cerebral hemisphere. The spheno-parietal sinus lies along the undersurface of the posterior border. Medial end of each posterior border projects backward as a prominent anterior clinoid process, which gives attachments to the following :

- anterior end of the free margin of the tentorium cerebelli;
- carotido-clinoid ligament, connecting with middle clinoid process;
- inter-clinoid ligament, extending between anterior and posterior clinoid processes.

The upper surface of lesser wing forms a part of the floor of anterior cranial fossa and is related to the orbital surface of the frontal lobe. The lower surface forms posterior part of the roof of orbit and presents the anterior opening of optic canal. Just outside the upper and medial margins of the optic canal it gives attachment to a part of common tendinous ring for the origins of the four recti muscles of eyeball. Outside the tendinous ring the lower surface provides separate origins of levator palpabrae superioris and more medially the superior oblique muscle of eyeball.

Superior orbital fissure

It is a retort-shaped cleft between the lesser and the greater wings.

Pterygoid processes

These extend vertically downwards from the junctions of the root of greater wings and the body. Each process consists of lateral and medial pterygoid plates which are separated behind from each other by a pterygoid fossa. Anterior surface of both plates is continuous and forms the posterior wall of pterygopalatine fossa which presents in the upper part the following three foramina from lateral to medial side with downward inclination: (i) foramen rotundum, (ii) anterior opening of pterygoid canal, (iii) palatino-vaginal or pharyngeal canal.

Posterior margin is also free and presents a small process near its centre for the attachment of pterygo-spinous ligament from the spine of sphenoid. lateral surface of the lateral plate forms the medial wall of infra-temporal fossa and provides origin to the lower head of lateral pterygoid muscle. Medial surface of the plate gives principal origin to medial pterygoid muscle. Therefore, the lateral pterygoid plate is a muscular plate.

The medial pterygoid plate is more elongated and presents anterior and posterior margins, lateral and medial surfaces. Anterior margin articulates with the posterior border of perpendicular plate of palatine bone. Posterior margin is free and presents in the lower part a hook-like process, the pterygoid hamulus, around the lateral side of which the tendon of the tensor veli palatini turns abruptly as the palatine aponeurosis. The tip of the hamulus gives attachment to the pterygo-mandibular raphe; the latter is attached below to the mandible behind the last molar tooth, and intervenes between the origins of buccinator in front and superior constrictor muscle of pharynx behind. Close to the hamulus the lower part of posterior border gives attachment to the upper part of superior constrictor muscle of pharynx along with bucco-pharyngeal and pharyngo-basilar fasciae. Traced above, the posterior border of medial plate forms a scaphoid fossa which provides principal origin of tensor veli palatini. A triangular projection of bone, processus tuberius, affects the middle of the posterior border and the notched area above the process lodges the medial end of the cartilagenous part of auditory tube, before the latter opens into the lateral wall of naso-pharynx.

Some important observations

- ***Fissures related to the bone:*** superior orbital and, inferior orbital fissures pterygo-maxillary fissures, and pterygoid fissures.
- ***Nerves related to the bone:*** Olfactory tracts above the jugum sphenoidale optic nerve in the optic canal; 3rd, 4th, 6th and three branches (lacrimal, frontal, naso-ciliary) of ophthalmic division of Vth cranial nerves in the superior orbital fissure; maxillary nerve (Vth cr.) through foramen rotundum: mandibular nerve (Vth cr.) and lesser pertosal nerve through foramen ovale; nervous spinosus in foramen spinosum; pterygoid nerve through the corresponding canal: chorda tympani nerve (VII cr.) medial to the sphenoidal spine; auriculo-temporal nerve lateral to the spine; pharyngeal nerve through palatino-vaginal canal.
- ***Venous sinuses related to the bone:*** cavernous sinuses on each side of the body: anterior and posterior intercavernous sinuses : spheno-palatine sinuses; middle meningeal sinuses.

OSSIFICATION

The tuberculum sellae divides the bone into pre - and post-sphenoidal parts; both parts are fused in the 7th or 8th months of intrauterine life.

Pre-sphenoidal part includes anterior part of the body and both lesser wings, and is ossified from six centres in cartilage: One for each lesser wing; two centres for the anterior part of the body, and one for each sphenoidal concha.

Post-sphenoidal part is ossified from eight centres: one for each greater wing ; the root of greater wing including pterygoid canal and foramen rotundum is ossified in cartilage; rest of the greater wing and lateral pterygoid plate are ossified from the same centre in membrane; two centres appear in cartilage for the posterior part of the body; one centre for each medial pterygoid plate in membrane, except the hamulus which is ossified in cartilage; one for each lingula in cartilage. At birth, the sphenoid consists of three pieces, the greater wing and pterygoid process on each side forming other two pieces. During the first year the pieces unite to form a single bone.

APPLIED ANATOMY

1. Premature synostosis between pre- and post-sphenoidal parts produces depression of the nasal bridge.
2. Abnormal growth of the pre-sphenoidal part produces separation of orbital cavities with hyper-telorism and a broad nasal bridge.

38
The Temporal Bones

The tubercle of the root of zygoma gives attachment to the lateral temporomandibular ligament.

The upper margin of the zygomatic arch is sharp and gives attachment to the downward extension of galea aponeurotica and more medially to temporal fascia. The lower margin is rough and gives origin to the masseter which extends also to the inner surface of the arch along the lower margin. (For further details see Norma lateralis).

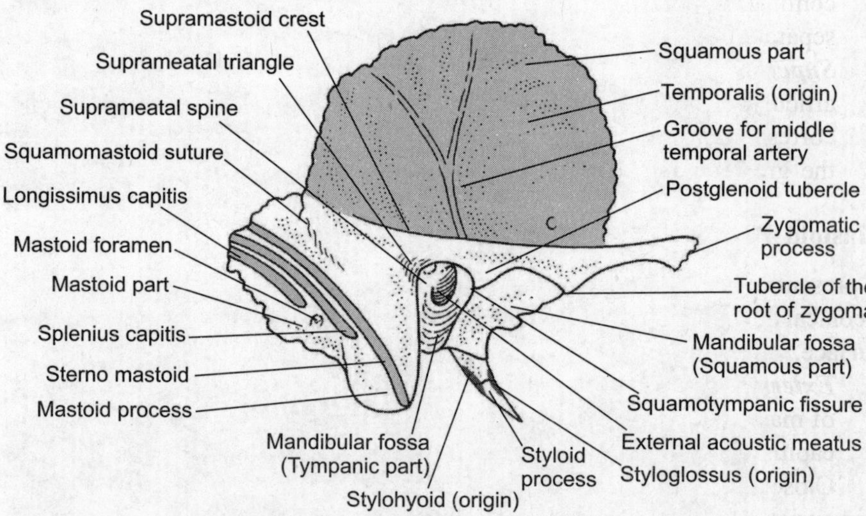

Fig. 38.1. Right temporal bone : External aspect.

MANDIBULAR FOSSA

It presents an articular area in front formed by the squamous part and a non-articular area behind formed by the tympanic part. The squamo-tympanic fissure intervenes between them. This fissure is subdivided by the down-turned edge of tegmen tympani from the petrous part into a petrotympanic fissure behind. and a petrosquamosal fissure in front.

The medial end of petrotympanic fissure transmits the following:

1. exit of the chorda tympani nerve (from facial) through its anterior canaliculus;
2. entry of the anterior tympanic branch of maxillary artery;
3. passage of the anterior ligament of malleus.

Articular part of the fossa including the articular eminence receives the head of the mandible separated by a fibro-cartilagenous articular disc and forms the synovial temporo-mandibular joint; the disc divides the joint into an upper menisco-temporal compartment and a lower menisco-mandibular compartment. The peripheral margin of the articular fossa, including the petrosquamosal fissure, gives attachment to the fibrous capsule of the joint.

The tympanic plate in the non-articular part of the fossa is separated from the joint capsule by a part of parotid gland.

- ***Internal (cerebral) surface*:** It is concave, marked by impressions for the gyri of the temporal lobe and presents grooves for the anterior and posterior divisions of middle meningeal vessels. This surface is continuous below with the anterior surface of the petrous part, often separated by traces of petrosquamosal suture.
- ***Superior border:*** It is convex, bevelled internally and overlaps for articulation with the middle third or more of the lower border of the corresponding parietal bone. Antero-inferior border. It articulates with the greater wing of the sphenoid.

Mastoid Part

It presents external and internal surfaces, superior and posterior borders, and a conical downward projection, the mastoid process, as an extension of external surface.

- ***External surface:*** It is rough and convex. Along with the outer surface of mastoid process provides attachments to sternocleidomastoid, splenius capitis and longissimus capitis from above downwards.

Close to the squamo-mastoid junction, occipital belly of occipito-frontalis and auricularis posterior muscles gain attachments.

A mastoid foramen is usually visible on this surface close to the occipito-mastoid suture. The foramen transmits an emissary vein connecting the sigmoid sinus with the posterior auricular vein, and a meningeal branch from the occipital artery.

- ***Internal surface:*** It is marked by a well-defined and curved sigmoid sulcus along its junction with the posterior surface of petrous part for the lodgement of sigmoid sinus. The floor of the sulcus is separated

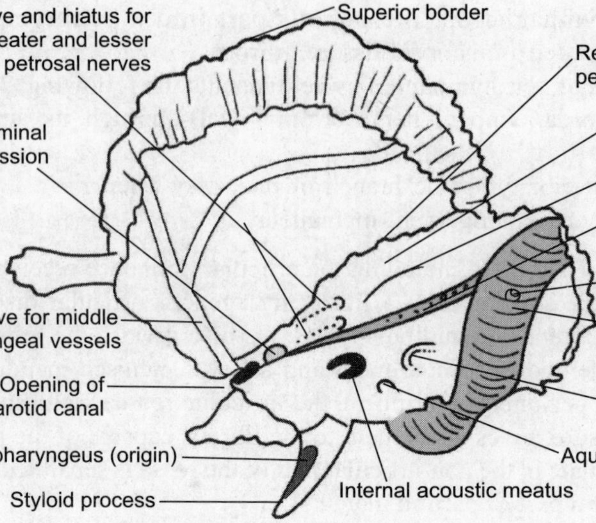

Fig. 38.2. The right temporal bone : Internal aspect.

from mastoid air cells by a thin plate of bone, and occasionally receives the inner opening of mastoid foramen.

- ***Superior border:*** It is serrated and articulates with the posterior one-third of lower border of parietal bone.
- ***Posterior border:*** It is serrated, articulates with the squamous part of occipital bone extending from lateral angle to the jugular process.
- ***Mastoid process:*** The inner surface presents a mastoid notch which gives origin to the posterior belly of digastric muscle. More medial to the notch lies a groove which runs upward for occipital artery.

The mastoid process is absent in the new born and appears at about second year, when the child holds the head upright by the pull of the sternocleidomastoid.

Tympanic Part

A curved plate of bone, situated below the squamous part and in front of the mastoid part. It presents anterior and posterior surfaces, and three borders—superior, inferior and lateral.

- ***Anterior surface:*** It forms the non-articular posterior part of mandibular fossa, and is related to a part of parotid gland.
- ***Posterior surface:*** is concave, and forms the anterior wall, floor and lower part of posterior wall of the bony part of external acoustic meatus.

- ***Superior border:*** It meets the squamous part separated by the squamo-tympanic fissure, which is subdivided in the medial part by the down-turned edge of tegmen tympani into petro-tympanic and petro-squamosal fissures (vide supra).
- ***Inferior border:*** It is thin, sharp and encroaches on the inferior surface of the .petrous part, where the border splits to enclose the root of styloid process of temporal bone as a sheath (vaginal process). The deep lamella of parotid fascia is attached along this border.
- ***Lateral border:*** It presents a curved ridge to form the lateral opening of the bony external meatus, where cartilagenous part of the meatus is attached. The posterior upturned end of lateral border is separated from the mastoid part by a tympano-mastoid fissure through which auricular branch of vagus nerve emerges.
- ***Petrous Part and Styloid Process:*** It is the most important part of the bone, pyramidal in shape and contains the labyrinth of the internal ear, mucous covered air-filled spaces of tympanic cavity (middle ear) along with mastoid antrum and bony part of auditory tube, and is traversed by the internal carotid artery and facial nerve lodging within their bony canals.

The petrous part presents a base, an apex, three surfaces—anterior, posterior and inferior, and three borders—anterior, superior and posterior.

- ***Base:*** It merges with the inner surface of the squamous and mastoid parts.
- ***Apex:*** It presents an irregular blunt area, projects forward and medially with an upward tilt, and forms the postero-lateral boundary of foramen lacerum. It bears the anterior opening of carotid canal for the intra-cranial entrance of internal carotid artery.
- ***Anterior surface:*** It is directed in front and above, and forms a part of the floor of the middle cranial fossa. The anterior surface presents the following features:
    - ***Trigeminal impression:*** It forms a shallow fossa close to the apex of the petrous part and postero-lateral to foramen lace rum. It lodges the trigeminal ganglion (the sensory ganglion of Vth cr. nerve) in a pouch of dura mater, the caevum trigeminale (Meckel's cave). The impression is continuous behind with a notch for the lodgement of sensory and motor roots of trigeminal nerve.

      Further behind the trigeminal impression and separated by a shallow depression that forms the roof of internal acoustic meatus, there lies an elevated area, the arcuate eminence; the latter is produced by the upward bulging of the anterior (superior) semicircular canal.

Tegmen tympani is a thin plate of bone which covers rest of the anterior surface of petrous part. It forms a common roof from behind forward of mastoid antrum, tympanic cavity and bony part of auditory tube. The down-turned edge of lateral part of tegmen tympani projects to divide the squamotympanic fissure into two parts (vide supra).

The tegmen tympani presents two foramina, lateral and medial. from each of which a faint groove runs antero-medially. The lateral foramen transmits lesser petrosal nerve (from glossopharyngeal); the medial foramen transmits greater petrosal nerve (from facial).

Posterior surface

It faces backward and upward, forms a part of the floor of posterior cranial fossa and displays three important features :

- ***Internal acoustic meatus:*** It is a bony canal—about 1 cm long. It transmits motor and sensory roots of facial nerve, further below the vestibulo-cochlear nerve, and the labyrinthine artery between and behind them.

Behind the internal meatus lies an oblique slit which leads upward to a bony canal, the aqueduct of vestibule. It lodges the saccus and ductus endolymphaticus filled with endolymph.The subarcuate fossa is an indistinct depression that intervenes between and above the aforesaid features. It lodges a process of dura mater and transmits some blood vessels. The sub-arcuate fossa is prominent in the newborn.

Inferior surface

It is irregular and appears in the exterior of the base of the skull, intervening between the greater wing of the sphenoid and basilar part of occipital bones. The inferior surface presents ten features from before backwards :

1. A quadrilateral area below the apex gives origin to the levator veli palatini; lateral part of the area forms the sulcus tubae together with the posterior margin of the greater wing of sphenoid and is related to the cartilagenous part of auditory tube.
2. Lower opening of the carotid canal for the passage of internal carotid artery, surrounded by a plexus of sympathetic nerves through the apex of petrous part in the posterior wall of foramen lacerum, which it crosses.
3. Jugular fossa is a deep depression for the accommodation of the superior bulb of internal jugular vein.
4. Tympanic canallculus for the tympanic branch of glossopharyngeal nerve is found in a bony ridge between the carotid canal and jugular fossa.

5. A triangular depression for inferior ganglion of glossopharyngeal nerve lies in front of jugular fossa and medial to the carotid canal. From the apex of depression a bony canal, the cochlear canaliculus, extends upward and transmits aqueduct of cochlea and some cochlear blood vessels. The aqueduct conveys perilymph which communicates with the C.S.F. of sub-arachnoid space, often separated by sieve-like fibrous membrane.
6. Lateral wall of jugular fossa presents one or more mastoid canaliculi for the auricular branch of vagus nerve; the latter leaves the bone through the tympano-mastoid fissure.
7. A rough jugular surface posteriorly articulates with the jugular process of occipital bone.
8. The sharp lower border of the tympanic plate encroaches on this surface and splits to enclose the root of the styloid process and acts as a sheath for the latter. The deep layer of parotid fascia is attached to the lower border and makes it sharp by the downward pull of the fascia.
9. The styloid process, about 2.5 cm long, extends downward and forward. The styloid process gives attachments to three muscles, two ligaments and is related to a number of important structures.
   – ***Muscles:***
   1. Styloglossus (supplied by hypoglossal nerve);
   2. stylohyoid (supplied by facial nerve);
   3. stylopharyngeus from medial surface of the base (supplied by glossopharyngeal nerve).

   – ***Ligaments:***
   1. Stylohyoid ligament, extending from the tip of styloid process to the lesser cornu of hyoid bone, is a remnant of second branchial arch in which the cartilage cells are absorbed and fibrous membrane persists as the ligament;
   2. stylomandibular ligament, extending from styloid tip to posterior border of ramus of mandible just above the angle of the mandible, is derived from the investing layer of deep cervical fascia as its splits to enclose the parotid gland.

   – ***Relations of styloid process:*** Laterally, overlapped by the parotid gland through which facial nerve and external carotid artery traverse. Medially, internal jugular vein behind, internal carotid artery in front and last four cranial nerves (9th, 10th, 11th and 12th) intervening between them.

   Note: The styloid process along with the 3 muscles and 2 ligaments (vide supra) may be described as the styloid apparatus.
10. Stylomastoid foramen lies midway between the styloid process and the mastoid process. It transmits the facial nerve and stylomastoid branch of posterior auricular artery.

Note : In the newborn the stylomastoid foramen lies at the surface of the bone due to lack of downward growth of the mastoid process. Therefore, surgical incision of sub-cutaneous abscess behind the pinna of ear in a child should be done with care to avoid injury to the facial nerve.

Anterior border

Medial part of the border articulates with the posterior margin of the greater wing of the sphenoid and forms the sulcus tubae on the undersurface of base of the skull (vide supra). The lateral part of anterior border joins with the squamous, part of temporal bone and presents two bony canals, upper and lower, at the site of their fusion. Both canals are separated by a bony partition, and extend backward and laterally to communicate with the anterior wall of tympanic cavity. The upper canal transmits tensor tympani muscle and the lower canal forms the bony dart of auditory tube.

Superior border

It is the longest border, intervenes between the floor of middle and posterior cranial fossae, and affords attachment to the lateral margin of tentorium cerebelli with a groove for the superior petrosal sinus. A trigeminal notch affects the superior border just lateral to the tip and below the attachment of tentorium cerebelli, for the passage of motor and sensory roots of trigeminal nerve; at the tip of the petrous part the upper border is crossed by abducent nerve below the petrosphenoid ligament.

Posterior border

Its medial part is articular and lateral part free. The medial part articulates with the basilar part of occipital bone and the groove between them on the cranial surface lodges the inferior petrosal sinus. Lateral part of the border forms the supero-lateral boundary of jugular foramen; a triangular notch affects this part of the border for the lodgement of inferior ganglion of glossopharyngeal nerve. (for jugular foramen see the norma basalis).

OSSIFICATION

- Squamous part is ossified in membrane from a single centre in the 8th week of intrauterine life.
- Petromastoid part is ossified in cartilage from multiple centres (as many as 14)
- Tympanic part : ossified in membrane in the 3rd foetal month.
- The styloid process is developed from the cartilage of the second

branchial arch and is ossified from two centres; upper or tympanohyal part before birth and lower or stylohyal part after birth.

The fusion of the above-mentioned four components takes place during the first post-natal year. (In some cases the tympanohyal and stylohyal parts of the styloid process may not fuse.)

Some observations on temporal bone: Three ear ossicles within the tympanic cavity—malleus, incus and stapes, ossify independently in cartilage during the 4th foetal month. Malleus and incus are developed from the dorsal end of first branchial arch, and stapes from the dorsal end of second branchial arch.

NOTE : Tympanic cavity, mastoid antrum, three ear ossicles and internal ear are of full adult size at birth.

39
The Zygomatic Bone

Paired bones form the prominence of the cheek. Externally: is somewhat diamond shaped in outline.

Surfaces: 3

1. lateral,
2. orbital
3. temporal

Processes: 2

1. frontal
2. temporal

Borders: 5

1. antero–superior
2. postero–superior
3. antero–Inferior
4. postero–Inferior
5. postero–medial.

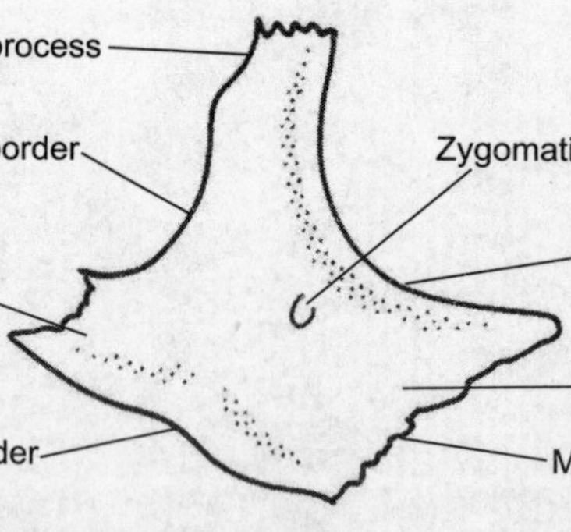

Fig. 39.1. Right zygomatic bone : Lateral view

1. – ***Lateral (facial) surface:*** convex, directed laterally and forward. Presents one or more foramina close to the orbital border for zygomatico-facial vessels and nerve. An oblique faint ridge seen on

this surface below the foramen: (i) anterior part of the ridge gives attachment to zygomaticus minor, (ii) its posterior part to zygomaticus major. It also provides a part of attachment to levator labii superioris.

– ***Orbital surface:*** Concave, smooth. Forms part of lateral wall and floor of the orbit, bears a zygomatico-orbital foramen which traverses the bone in a Y-shaped canal ; one limb of the canal appears on the lateral, surface for the passage of zygomatico-facial vessels and nerve, and the other limb appears on the temporal surface for zygomatico-temporal vessels and nerve.

2. The orbital surface extend along the frontal process of the bone, and presents within the orbital opening and 1 cm below the fronto-zygomatic suture, a Whitnall's tubercle, which gives attachment to:
   1. lateral palpebral ligament
   2. check ligament of rectus lateralis,
   3. suspensory ligament of eye ball
   4. the aponeurosis of levator palpebrae superioris.
3. ***Temporal surface:*** directed backward and medially, rough and articular in the anterior part, and smooth and concave in the posterior part. Anterior part articulates with the zygomatic process of maxilla. Posterior part forms the anterior wall of temporal and infra-temporal fossae and presents one or more zygomatico temporal foramina.
   – ***Frontal process*** – thick upward projection. Its upper end articulates with the zygomatic process of frontal bone suture. Postero-medial margin of the frontal process articulates with the lateral border of the orbital surface of the great wing of the sphenoid. The strong frontal process acts as a line of buttress for dispersion of force of impact to the frontal bone during mastication by the molar and premolar teeth.
   – **Temporal process**– extends backward and the serrated end joins with the zygomatic process of temporal bone to complete the zygomatic arch.

BORDERS

1. ***Antero-superior (orbital) border*** - concave, smooth and forms infero-lateral margin of orbit.
2. ***Postero-superior border*** - forms an italic "f" shaped sharp border and presents a marginal tubercle below the fronto-zygomatic suture. Traced above, it is continuous with the posterior border of the zygomatic process of frontal bone, and below with the upper margin of the zygomatic arch. Temporal fascia is attached along the entire border.
3. ***Antero-inferior border*** - articulates with maxilla.

4. ***Postero-inferior border*** - rough, continuous with lower margin of zygomatic arch, gives attachment to masseter.
5. ***Postero-medial border*** - It articulates with the lateral border of orbital surface of greater wing of the sphenoid in the upper part and with the maxilla in the lower part; sometimes a notch intervenes between them to form the lateral end of inferior orbital fissure.

Side determination of zygomatic bone : place the long and thick frontal process above, italic letter "f" shaped border behind and above, and the convex lateral surface determines the side of the bone.

OSSIFICATION

8th week ossifies in membrane from a single centre (in jejunum more than 1-2 centre) which appears in the 8th week of intrauterine life.

HISTOLOGY

Tables for Identification of Cells and Tissues

TABLE. Showing cytoplasmic organelles and inclusions

Organelles		**Inclusions**	
Names	**Functions**	**Names**	**Examples**
1. Ribosomes	Protein Synthesis	**1. Stored food**	glycogen, fat
2. Membranous organelles			
Cell membrane	Selective permeability	**2. Secretion granules or globules**	insulin
endoplasmic reticulum	protein synthesis		
mitochondria	cell respiration, metabolism	**3. Pigments**	
		exogenous	vegetable pigments *carotene* lipochrome dust, coal and silica minerals *silver, lead*
lysosomes (suicide bags)	dissolution of cells		
3. Centrosphere and centriole	cell division	***endogenous***	haemoglobin melanin
4. Fibrils, filaments and tubules			

TABLE. Showing chemical nature and staining characteristics of various cell components

Cell components	**Physical constituents**	**Chemical nature**	**Staining characteristics**
1. Nucleus	Chromatin	**DNA**	Purple-blue with haematoxylin (basophilia)
	Nucleolus	**RNA**	–do–
2. Cytoplasmic organelles	Ground substance	**Protein**	Pink-red with eosin (acidophilia or eosinophilia)
	Mitochondria	**Lipid protein complex**	Blue with Janus green B, Red with acid-fuchsin.
	Centrioles	**Protein**	Rarely seen in haematoxylin and eosin
	Chromophilic substance (ribosomes and endoplasmic reticulum)	**RNA**	Same as nucleus
	Fibrils	**Protein**	Special methods, argyrophilic
mitochondria	cell respiration, metabolism	**3. Pigments**	
3. Cytoplasmic inclusions.	Lipids	**Fats**	Blackened by osmium tetroxide (osmiophilia), negative image in haematozylin and eosin, removed by solvents).
	Zymogen	**Protein**	Red with eosin (eosinophilic)
	Mucigen Glycogen	**Carbohydrate**	Unstained in routine haematoxylin and wosin, negative image, Red to purple with periodic acid Schiff (PAS) stain.

TABLE. Chief distribution of simple epithelial subtypes

Squamous	Cuboidal	Columnar
1. Terminal and respiratory bronchioles and air sacs Nucleus	1. Germinal epithelium of ovary	1. Lining of alimentary canal from stomach to rectum
2. Body cavities (mesothelium)	2. Thyroid follicles	2. Gall bladder
3. Cardivascular and lymphatic system (endothelium)	3. Choroid plexus of brain ventricles	3. Small bronchi and large bronchioles
4. Smallest ducts of many glands	4. Pigment-epithelium of retina	4. Uterine tubes and uterus (in part) *ciliated columnar epithelium* is found in : a) Ependyma. b) endometrium of uterus (in part) c) uterine tubes (in part)
5. Descending limb of Henle's loop in kidney	5. Excretory ducts of some glands	2. Gall bladder
6. Mesenchymal epithelium lining cavities in connective tissue	2. Thyroid follicles	2. Gall bladder

TABLE 25. Showing the features of these sub-types of simple epithelia

	Squamous epithelium	Cuboidal epithelium	Columnar epithelium
1. Nucleus			
Shape	Flattened	Rounded DNA	Elongated or oval Basal
Distribution	Often missed in a number of cells.	Central	
Cells	Have a narrow rim of cytoplasm.	Have almost equal length and breadth	Have length more than the breath.

Table-27. Showing Differential Diagnosis of Stratified Squamous Epithelium

	Stratified Squamous Epithilium	Transitional Epithilium	Pseudostratified Epithilium
Surface cells	Flattened scale-like	Umbrella, baloon or dome dome-shaped. About 6 layers or less deep	Columnar
Number of layers (rows) of nuclei	Usually more than 8 layers		Deceptive appearance of stratification. All cells reach the basement membrane.
Nuclei	Occur in all layers. Flattened towards surface.	Occur in all layers. Surface layer possesses more globular than flattened nuclei.	Nuclei are of several types. Those at the base are small and dark. Those near surface are larger and paler. The majority lie below the middle of the epithelium.
Basal line of epithelium	Papillated	Not papillated	Not papillated

TABLE-28. Showing Differential Diagnosis of Pseudostratified Epithelium.

	Pseudostratified Epithelium	**Stratified Columnar Epithelium**
Surface	Columnar. All touch basal membrane.	Columnar. Do not touch basal membrane.
Basal cells	Not columnar. Do not extend to the free surface.	May appear cuboidal.
Morphology of nuclei	Of several types. Those at the base are small and dark. Those nearer the surface are larger and paler.	Compact and avoid, single type of nuclei forming a nearly straight row.
Basal nuclei	Irregularly arranged.	Form more or less a straight row.
Vertical extent of nuclei	The majority of nuclei lie well below the middle level of the total layer.	Nuclear portion comprises three fourth to four fifth of the entire epithelial layer.

TABLE-29. Showing Distinction Between Collagenous, Elastic, and Reticular Fibres

	Collagenous	**Elastic**	**Reticular**
Occurence	In bundles, parallel fibres bundles are wide e.g tendons.	Always occur singly e.g ligaments.	Anastomosing fibres (network)
Location of cells	Located at periphery of bundles of fibres.	Cells located between individual fibres.	Satellate cells, whose processes form delicate reticulum.
Numbers of cells	Few, wing shaped.	Cells more.	Many, star like.
Nuclei	Relatively long, dark staining with squared ends, resembling a series of dashes. Nuclei farther apart.	Shorter, more oval, less deeply staining. Nuclei lie close together.	Nuclei irregularly distributed.
Cross section *Connective tissue septa*	Fibres bundles distinct. Connective tissue septa very distinct.	Appears more homogenous, septa fewer and less distinct.	——
Special staining	Mallory stain gives *Blue colour.*	Orcein and resorcin fuchsin stains *purple black.*	Silver-staining renders fibres *Black.*
Relationship with lymphocytes	——	——	Always many lymphocytes caught in meshwork.

TABLE-30. Showing features of distinction between the three types of muscle fibres, both in transverse and longitudinal sections.

	Smooth muscle	Skeltal muscle	Cardiac muscle
Transverse section (T.S.)	Much smaller is size.	Largest in size.	Larger in size.
	Show wide size variation	Fair uniformity in size of any given muscle.	Moderate variation in size.
	They lack any visible stippling	Appears as plainly visible dots.	Show fibrils as visible as visible dots
	Nuclei centrally located.	Nuclei are in the peripheral part	Nuclei centrally located.
	Largest nuclei relative to fibre diametre	Smallest nuclei relative to fibre diametre	———
	Smooth muscle packed tightly with no obvious tissue fibres between them.	Skeletal muscle fibres embedded in connective tissue called endomysium	Cardiac muscle fibres embedded in connective tissue.
Longitudinal section (L.S.)	Seen as relatively small spindles which are unstriped.	Very large solitary bands seen strongly striped.	Coarse and branched network are seen as weakly striped.
	Nuclei slender and more elaborate than in other two types.	Many nuclei are seen.	Nuclei are ovoid in shape.

TABLE-31. Differential diagnosis of the smooth muscle fibres and the connective tissue.

	Smooth muscle fibres	Connective tissue
1. Nuclei	Lie inside muscle fibres.	Lie between connective tissue fibres.
2. Cytoplasm	Darker stained with eosin ribosomes of muscle cytoplasm take haematoxylin (give purlish tinct).	Lighter stained with eosin.
3. Other kinds of cells	No other kind of cells occur between the muscle fibres within a bundle of sheet.	Other kinds of cells occur between connective tissue fibres.
4. Masson's trichrome stain	Stained red	Stained blue.

TABLE-32. Showing difference between spleen, lymph nodes and thymus

	Spleen	**Lymphnode**	**Thymus**
Cortex	Absent	Present	Present
Medulla	Absent	Present	Present
Characterisitic features	Capsule shows the smooth muscle fibres. Trabeculae present. Lymph nodules show central arteriole.	Underneath the capsule, a subcapsular sinus is present. Trabeculae present.	Capsule is thin. Cortex is dense peripheral part. Medulla is lightly stained central portion.
Transverse section (T.S.)	Dense lymphoid tissue (white pulp) and numerous R.B.C. (red pulp) can be seen.	Cortex shows lymphatic nodules.	Thymocytes form parenchyma. Hassal's corpuscles found in meddula.

TABLE-33. Showing distinguishing features between various types of tonsils

	Palatine	**Lingual tonsil**	**Nasopharyngeal tonsil**
1. Epithelium	Stratified squamous.	Stratified squamous.	Pseudostratified columnar.
2. Crypts	Deep, branching and longer.	Pit-like.	Pit-like.
3. Lymph nodules	Present beneath epithelium and around crypts.	Present around crypts only.	Present around bases of crypts.
4. Capsule	Thick and well-defined.	....	....

TABLE-38. Showing examples of exocrine, endocrine and exo-endocrine glands in the human body

Exocrine glands	Endocrine glands	Exo-endocrine glands
1. Lacrimal 2. Parotid 3. Submandibular 4. Sublingual 5. Sebaceous 6. Sweat 7. Mammary 8. Meibomian 9. Glands of Zeis 10. Kidney 11. Prostate 12. Seminal Vesicle 13. Goblet cells (Unicellular gland) 14. Greater vestibular (Bartholin's gland) 15. Bulbourethral (Cowper's gland)	1. Hypophysis 2. Parathyroid 3. Adrenal (Both cortex & medulla) 4. Placenta 5. Thymus? 6. Pineal body?	1. Pancreas **Exocrine-**pancreatic acini **Endocrine-**islets of Langerhans 2. Thyroid **Exocrine-**secretions coming into lumen of vesicles for storage. **Endocrine-**secretion into blood capillaries, and secretion of calcitonin. 3. Testis **Exocrine-**cytogenic excretion of sperms into ducts of testis **Endocrine-**intestitial cells of Leydig. 4. Ovary **Exocrine-**cytogenic excretion of ova into peritoneal cavity. **Endocrine-**granulosa cells and corpus luteum. 5. Liver **Exocrine-**secretion of bile. **Exocrine-** secretion of glucose etc.

TABLE-40. Distinguish features between serous and mucos acini in the salivary glands

Lumen	Very small (difficult to be seen)	Prominent (easily seen)
Cytoplasm of lining cells	Basophilic at the base of cells. Eosinophilic toward apex due to zymogen granules.	Less basophilia at the bases. Mucigen granules present between the nucleus and apex of mucous cells, do not stain well with H/E. Hence appear pale and vacuolated.
Nuclei	Usually oval or spherical (not pressed against bases of the cell)	Usually appear flattened and pressed against the base of cells.

TABLE-49. Showing difference between the adrenal gland and corpus luteum

Features	Adrenal gland	Corpus luteum
Capsule	Connective tissue capsule surrounds the glands.	Connective tissue capsule is missing.
Cortex	Is divided into zona-glomerulosa (short columnar cells arranged in ovoid, C or U shaped groups), zona-fasciculata (arranged in palisade like fashion at right angles to the surface), and zona reticularis (consisting of cells arranged in branching and anastomosing cords).	It shows large polyhedral lutein cells, with often indistinct cell walls, arranged in irregular masses.
Medulla	It is more loosely arranged central portion which stains darker with H/E than cortex. Irregular cells, arranged in rounded groups or short cords, show chromaffin reaction as they contain specific granules in their cytoplasm. Large veins are also seen.	Shows numerous large folds surrounding a central cavity which is filled with loose connective tissue. On its outer side large polyhedral cells are also seen.

TABLE-60. Differentiating features between artery and vein of the same size

Features	Artery	Vein
Lumen	Smaller	Larger.
Wall	Thicker and more rigid	Thinner wall
Shape	Held relatively better, less likely to collapse	More likely to collapse.
Elastic & muscular tissue	More.	Less.
Tunica media	Thicker.	Inconspicuous.
Tunica adventitia	Less developed	Thickest.
Internal elastic lamina	Distinct.	Not distinct.
All the three coats	Clearly differetiated.	Lack clear differentiation
Post mortem contraction	Stronger, hence leaves no blood in the lumen.	Weaker, leaves blood in the lumen.
Valves	Not present	Present in some veins.
Lymphatics	Absent in the wall of arteries.	Abundant in the wall of veins.

TABLE: Showing a comparison of the chief features of the three types of connective tissue fibres

		Collagenous (White)	Elastic (Yellow)	Reticular (Argyrophilic)
1.	**Terminology**	Because they consist of an albuminous substance-collagen. Termed white owing to lack of colour (L.colla, glue).	Because they consist of a protein-elastin. Termed yellow owing to their distinctive colour.	Because they are disposed in tiny network (L. reticularis, a little net). Termed argyrophilic owing to their impregnation with silver.
2.	**Formation**	Produced by fibroblasts. Soluble Collagen (tropocollagen) which is secreted by the cell condenses in mucopolysaccharides to form fibrils.	Little is known of the exact formation. Some regard elastic fibres as being derived from collagen.	Similar to that of collagenous fibres.
3.	**Distribution**	Tendons, ligaments and aponeuroses. vocal cords, ligamentum flavum and ligamentum nuchae.	Blood vessels, distensible viscera, marrow, liver, lungs and spleen.	Framework of lymph gland, bone
4.	**Morphology**	Broad, somewhat wavy bundles of fibrils, bound together by cement substance and limiting membrane. Do not branch. Thickness 1-100 U or more.	Fine the threads. Branch and anastomose freely with each other. Thickness 10-12 U.	Very fine fibrils in a network. In thickness these are much thinner. Diameter about 0.01 U.
5.	**Physicochemicl properties**			
(i)	Refreactive index.	Low (appear dark).	High (appear bright)	Intermediate.
(ii)	Resistance to chemical change	Fair.	perhaps most resistant material in body.	Not so resistant.
(iii)	Action of Acid pepsin.	Easily digested.	Slowly digested (pancreatic elastase digests it)	More resistant to peptic digestion than collagenous fibres.
6.	**Effect of boiling with water.**	Form gelatin	Not affected by hot or cold water, dilute acids or alkalies or by gastric juice.	Form reticulin.
7.	**Functions**	Principally act as binding material. Afford great tensile strength.	Afford elasticity to blood vessels. Ageing causes arteriosclerosis.	Supply a yielding matrix for cells and hold them in place.

Table continued

8.	**Staining characteristics**			
i	H/E staining	Pink	Usually not coloured	Faintly pink.
ii	Orcein and Resorcinfuchscin	Not stained.	Purple black	Not stained.
iii	Silver technique	Not blackened (cola-yellow or brown)	Usually not blackened	Specially blackened
iv	PAS(periodic acid schiff technique)	Slightly PAS positive.	PAS negative (sometimes positive)	Strongly PAS positive.

TABLE: Showing comparison between three types of cartilages.

		Hyaline (glass-like cartilage)	**Fibrous** (white fibro-cartilage)	**Elastic** (yellow fibro-cartilage)
1.	**Distribution**	1. Sternal ends of ribs. 2. Articular ends of long bones. 3. Cartilages of nose. 4. Some of the laryngeal cartilages (thyoid and cricoid). 5. Cartilages of trachea and bronchi. 6. Whole of the foetal skeleton.	(Where tensile strength is desired) 1. Intervertiberal disc. 2. Articular disc. 3. Lining tendon grooves.	(Where support and flexibility is required) 1. Pinna (external ear). 2. Lining of external acoustic meatus and auditory tube. 3. Epiglottis. 4. Corniculate cartilages. 5. Lining tendon grooves.
2.	**Colour**	Opalescent bluish-tint transluscent.	Opaque.	Yellow, more opaque than hyaline.
3.	**Texture**	———	Firm	Flexible and elastic.
4.	**Perichondrium**	Present, composed of firm fibrous tissue.	Absent.	An ensheathing perichondrium is present.
5.	**Cartilage cells**	Large (40 U), show marked shrinkage vacuolation and distortion when fixed. Occur singly in young cartilage, in groups (cell nests) later on.	Sparse, occur as single or in groups and row.	Similar to hyaline, occur singly or in groups.
6.	**Matrix**	Homogenous, basophilic. Actually it is stiff and gelatinous substance permeated by a felt work of fine collagenous fibrills.	Visible in near vicinity of cells. Cartilage capsules are deeply stained. Coarse collagen fibres rae present. These may interweave.	In addition there is a mesh work of elastic fibres. Fibres are thicker and more closely packed. They are irregularly branched.
7.	**Functions**	Principally act as binding material. Afford great tensile strength.	Afford elasticity to blood vessels. Ageing causes arteriosclerosis.	Supply a yielding matrix for cells and hold them in place.
8.	**Staining characteristics**			
i	H/E staining	Pink	Usually not coloured	Faintly pink.
ii	Orcein and Resorcinfuchscin	Not stained.	Purple black	Not stained.
iii	Silver technique	Not blackened (cola-yellow or brown)	Usually not blackened	Specially blackened
iv	PAS(periodic acid schiff technique)	Slightly PAS positive.	PAS negative (sometimes positive)	Strongly PAS positive.

TABLE-37

	Oesophagus	Pharynx (oral and laryngeal)	Urinary bladder
1. Mucosa			
Epithelium	Non-keratinized stratified squamous.	Soft staratified squamous.	Transitional.
Cell Layers	About 25	20-25	6-8
Lamina propria	Shows tall papillae which indent the epithelium.	Shows small papillae which indent the epithelium.	No papillae. Junction with epithelium is smooth.
Muscular mucosae	Thicker than any where else in body.	Absent.	Absent.
2. Sub-mucosa			
Elastic tissue layer	Absent.	Present as a distinct layer.	Some elastic fibres are seen.
Glands	Mucous glands seen in submucosa.	Few small mucous glands are seen.	Absent.
3. Muscularis	Both are inner circullar and outer longitudinal muscle layers are thick. Upper and middle1/3 shows straited and the lower 1/3 shows smooth muscle fibres.	Inner longitudinal and outer circular layers of striated muscle fibres (note the reversed order)	Two to three loosely arranged layers. Inner longitudinal, middle circular and outer longitudinal layer of smooth muscle fibres.
4. Adventitia fibrosa or serosa	Loose fibrous layer, in abdomen it is partly covered by a serosa.	Thin fibrous layer.	Thin fibrous layer (on upper surface of bladder is peritoneum).

TABLE-52. Differential diagnosis of the pharynx, tongue, urinary bladder and uterus.

Features	Pharynx	Tongue	Urinary bladder
Epithelium	Stratified squamous epithelium.	Thick layer of stratified squamous epithelium. Upper surface studded with projections. Filiform, fungiform and vallate papillae are seen.	Folded surface. Transitional epithelium. 2 to 4 layers in distended bladder and 6 to 8 layers in the contracted bladder. Pits seen in epithelial surface.
Lamina proria	Fairly dense connective tissue containing both elastic and collagenous fibres.	Composed of connective tissue, which forms the core of the papillae.	Connective the tissue of lamina propria and sub mucosa blended.
Muscular Layer	Striated muscle not in definite layers. Mucous or seromucous glands may penetrate the muscle layer (inner longitudinal and outer circular).	Comples musculateure, although bundles of striated muscle fibres interlace in all directions. Three distinct planes:vertical, transverse and longitudinal can be differentiated.	Rather thick muscle coat, made up of three layers of smooth muscle. Outer longitudinal, middle circular and inner longitudinal; but muscle layers distinctly seperated.

Index